Clinical Skills for Assistive Personnel

Sheila A. Sorrentino, RN, PhD

Curriculum Consultant
Normal, Illinois

with 176 illustrations

Mosby

St. Louis Baltimore Boston Carlsbad Chicago Minneapolis New York Philadelphia Portland
London Milan Sydney Tokyo Toronto

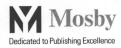
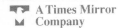

Publisher: Sally Schrefer
Senior Editor: Susan R. Epstein
Associate Developmental Editor: Jerry Schwartz
Project Manager: John Rogers
Project Specialist: Kathleen L. Teal
Design Coordinator: Renée Duenow
Manufacturing Manager: Linda Ierardi
Cover Design: David A. Scott

Printed in the United States of America
Composition by Graphic World, Inc.
Printing/binding by Von Hoffman Press

Mosby, Inc.
11830 Westline Industrial Drive
St. Louis, Missouri 63146

International Standard Book Number 0-3230-0074-6

98 99 00 01 02 / 9 8 7 6 5 4 3 2 1

To Uncle Seth and Aunt Theresa,
my godparents

Sheila A. Sorrentino

Reviewers

Jane Taylor Duncan, BSN
Department Chair
Gaston College
Gastonia, North Carolina

Phyllis J. Nichols, RN
Patient Care Technician Instructor
Tucson College
Tucson, Arizona

Carol S. Wells, RN, BSN, MS
Nurse Educator
St. Vincent's Medical Center
Jacksonville, Florida

Denise R. York, RNC, MS, MEd
Assistant Professor
Columbus State Community College
Columbus, Ohio

Acknowledgments

No book is written and published by the efforts of one person. The planning, manuscript development and review, and production processes involve the insights, talents, and contributions of many individuals. I am especially grateful to:

Carol Miller, Employment Specialist at OSF St. Joseph Medical Center in Bloomington, Illinois for helping me secure job descriptions, employee handbooks, and other information.

Jane DeBlois, Education Coordinator at OSF St. Joseph Medical Center for sharing materials and information, reviewing art, and for helping me problem solve.

Becky Powell, Pam Ward, Rita Schlomer, Kathy Coyle, and Joan Stralow at OSF St. Joseph Medical Center for sharing information and providing clinical expertise.

Pat Nolan, Patient Education Coordinator at Genesis Medical Center in Davenport, Iowa, for sharing information.

Wendy Woith, formerly Director of Clinical Practice at BroMenn Regional Medical Center in Bloomington, Illinois, for sharing competency materials.

Anne Perry and Pat Potter, authors of *Clinical Nursing Skills and Techniques* (fourth edition), for sharing galleys with me. Their sections on "Delegation Considerations" were invaluable in resolving content issues.

Bernie Gorek, co-author of *Mosby's Textbook for Long-Term Care Assistants* (third edition) and Director of Nursing Services and Community Health Services at Bonell Good Samaritan Center in Greeley, Colorado, for her insights and advice.

Jack Tandy of St. Louis for his artwork.

Rick Brady of Reva, Maryland, for his photography.

The staff at Anne Arundel Medical Center in Annapolis, Maryland for their patience and help during photography sessions.

Jane Duncan, Phyllis Nichols, Carol Wells, and Denise York for reviewing the manuscript and for their candor and suggestions. They have contributed to the thoroughness and accuracy of this book.

Connie Leinicke, freelance editor in St. Louis, for helping with the manuscript review process and for securing permissions.

The people at Mosby, especially Suzi Epstein, Betty Hazelwood, Kathy Teal, and Alison Harrison. Alison brought order and direction to this project before turning it over to the capable and talented hands of Suzi Epstein. Suzi provided me with valuable insights, guidance, and support. She also injected a sense of humor at the right times. Betty Hazelwood was amazing as a copy editor. Her attention to detail enhanced the quality of this book. Kathy Teal's excellent page layout made the proofreading and production process easy and pleasant.

To all those who contributed to this effort in any way, I am sincerely grateful.

Sheila A. Sorrentino

Preface to the Instructor

The rising cost of health care has forced hospitals and other health care facilities to restructure the delivery of nursing care and other patient care services. Of the many strategies that emerged, the return to a nursing staff mix and patient-focused care affected the traditional nursing assistant role. New titles and new job descriptions developed. Patient care technician, health care assistant, nurse extender, and patient care attendant are some titles that attempt to describe the expanding role of unlicensed assistive personnel. Job descriptions include complex nursing tasks and activities such as wound care, catheterizations, suctioning, and assisting with IV therapy. Phlebotomy and obtaining an ECG are examples of cross-training for purposes of moving hospital services from departments to the bedside.

Clinical Skills for Assistive Personnel was created in response to the teaching and learning needs that result when assistive personnel assume tasks and activities beyond the traditional nursing assistant role. Although much controversy exists about the expanding role of assistive personnel, an ethical and legal imperative exists to provide such individuals with the necessary education and training for safe and effective functioning. Inherent in safe functioning is the need to understand the legal aspects of the role and delegation principles.

CONTENT ISSUES

Unlike nursing assistant education which has minimum standards set by the Omnibus Budget Reconciliation Act of 1987, no standardization exists for the expanded role of assistive personnel. Functions vary from hospital to hospital within the same community. Assistive personnel in the same hospital may have different titles and functions in different nursing areas. Some hospitals are more liberal than others in what assistive personnel are allowed to do. State guidelines vary. Some states issued advisory opinions based on their nurse practice acts while others enacted legislation specific to the role. Thus, content issues were created.

In deciding what to present in *Clinical Skills for Assistive Personnel,* a multitude of resources were studied. The content in this book reflects a critical analysis and synthesis of information collected from:

- State laws, guidelines, and advisory opinions
- State curricula
- Job descriptions
- The current literature
- Research studies
- Training programs developed by hospitals, educational institutions, and associations
- Focus groups
- Personal interviews

TRENDS

Several trends emerged in the process of resolving content issues and were accommodated in the organization and development of the book.

- Nursing assistant education and training is often a requisite for the expanded assistive role. Therefore, *Mosby's Textbook for Nursing Assistants* (fourth edition) serves as the foundation for this book. *Clinical Skills for Assistive Personnel* builds upon nursing assistant education and training and presents new knowledge and skills.

- Other than the umbrella title of "unlicensed assistive personnel" or "UAP," no universal title exists to describe the role under discussion. Although it serves a legal purpose, many individuals interviewed consider "unlicensed" to have negative connotations. Additionally, New Hampshire does license nursing assistants. For these reasons, using "unlicensed" was deemed undesirable. Therefore, "assistive personnel" is the term used in the title and throughout the book in referring to persons who assist nurses in providing patient care.

- The need for good "work ethics" was a consistent theme among individuals participating in Mosby's market research. Thus, an entire section in Chapter 1 was developed on behavior in the workplace.

- Effective delegation was a common theme in the literature and is a major focus of the National Council of State Boards of Nursing. RNs must make responsible delegation decisions. However, assistive personnel must decide whether or not to accept or refuse a delegated task or activity. Delegation is discussed in Chapter 1. Throughout the book the student is cautioned to perform a task or activity only if certain conditions are met.

FEATURES, DESIGN, AND PHILOSOPHICAL APPROACH

In essence, *Clinical Skills for Assistive Personnel* is a supplement to *Mosby's Textbook for Nursing Assistants* (fourth edition). Therefore, the features, design elements, and philosophical approach are consistent with *Mosby's Textbook for Nursing Assistants*.

Readability

On the advice of a reading specialist, the design features the following:

- Key terms with definitions appear at the beginning of each chapter and are in bold print throughout the text. The definition is presented in the text.

- Procedure boxes are divided into pre-procedure, procedure, and post-procedure steps. Labeling and color gradients differentiate the sections.

- Review questions are found at the end of each chapter. They are followed by the page number where the answers are listed.

- Boxes are used to list principles, rules, signs and symptoms, and other information. The boxes present an efficient way for instructors to highlight content and provide useful study guides for students.

- Bullets are used for each item in a list rather than numbering.

Values

The importance of caring and treating the patient as a *person* is an important message throughout this book. The words "person" or "persons" are used whenever possible in reference to the individual to instill the value that the recipient of care is more than a "patient."

Other values and principles retained from *Mosby's Textbook for Nursing Assistants* and its previous editions include:

- Safe functioning within the legal limits of the assistive role while recognizing that such limits may vary among states.

- Respect for the person and recognition that each person is a physical, social, psychological, and spiritual human being with basic needs.

- The importance of personal choice and dignity of person.

- The need for assistive personnel to be aware of and understand their work environment and the individuals in that environment.

- That understanding body structure and function and normal growth and development are helpful for developing desirable attitudes toward individuals and for performing nursing skills safely and competently.

Added Features

Age-specific competency requirements by the Joint Commission on Accreditation of Healthcare Organizations (JCAHO) were also considered when developing this book. So were the special considerations inherent in home care. Therefore, *Focus on Children, Focus on Older Persons,* and *Focus on Home Care* appear in green shading throughout the book as appropriate. The *Focus on . . .* segments serve to provide insight into the needs, considerations, and special circumstances of children and older persons and to that of home care.

I hope that this book will serve you and your students well. My intent is to provide you and your students with the information needed to teach and learn safe and effective care during this time of dynamic change in health care.

Sheila A. Sorrentino, RN, BSN, MA, MSN, PhD

Preface to the Student

This book was designed for you. It was designed to help you learn. The book is a useful resource as you gain experience and expand your knowledge. This preface gives some study guidelines and helps you use the book. When giving a reading assignment do you read from the first page to the last page without stopping? How much do you remember? You will learn more if you use a study system. A useful study system has these steps:

- Survey or preview
- Question
- Read and record
- Recite and review

PREVIEW

Before you start a reading assignment, preview or survey the assignment. This gives you an idea of what the assignment covers. It also helps you recall what you already know about the subject. Carefully look over the assignment. Preview the chapter title, headings, subheadings, and terms or ideas in bold print or italics. Also survey the objectives, key terms, first paragraph, boxes and the summary and review questions at the end of the chapter. Previewing only takes a few minutes. Remember, previewing helps you become familiar with the material.

QUESTION

After previewing, you need to form questions to answer while you read. Questions should relate to what might be asked on a test or how the information applies to giving care. Use the title, headings, and subheadings to form questions. Avoid questions that have one word answers. Questions that begin with what, how, or why are helpful. While reading, you may find that a question does not help you study. If so, just change the question. Remem-ber, questioning sets a purpose for reading. So changing a question only makes this step more useful.

READ AND RECORD

Reading is the next step. Reading is more productive after determining what you already know and what you need to learn. Read to find answers to your questions. The purpose of reading is to:

- Gain new information
- Connect the new information to what you know already

Break the assignment into smaller parts. Then answer your questions as you read each part. Also, mark important information. The information can be marked by underlining, highlighting, or making notes. Underlining and highlighting remind you what you need to learn. You need to go back and review the marked parts later. Making notes results in more immediate learning. When making notes, you write down important information in the margins or in a notebook. Use words and summary statements that will jog your memory about the material.

After reading the assignment, you need to remember the information. To remember the material, you must work with the information. This step involves organizing information into a study guide. Study guides have many forms. Diagrams or charts help show relationships or steps in a process. Much of the information in this text is organized in this manner to help you learn. Note taking in outline format is also very useful. The following is a sample outline:

1. Main heading
   a. Second level
   b. Second level
      i. Third level
      ii. Third level
2. Main heading

RECITE AND REVIEW

Finally, recite and review. Use your notes and the study guides. Answer the questions you formed earlier. Also answer any other questions that came up during the reading and the review questions at the end of the chapter. Answer all questions out loud (recite).

Reviewing is more about *when* to study rather than *what* to study. You already determined what to study during the preview, question, and reading steps. The best times to review the material are right after the first study session, one week later, and regularly before a test, midterm, or final exam.

The editors at Mosby and I want you to enjoy learning. We also want you to enjoy your work. You and your work are important. You and the care you give may be bright spots in a person's day. This book was also designed to help you study. Special design features are decribed on the next pages.

Objectives tell you what will be presented and what you need to learn.

Key terms are the important words and phrases in the chapter. Definitions are given for each term. The key terms introduce you to the chapter content. They are also useful study guides.

Bolded type is used to highlight the key terms in the text. You again see the key term and read its definition. This helps reinforce your learning.

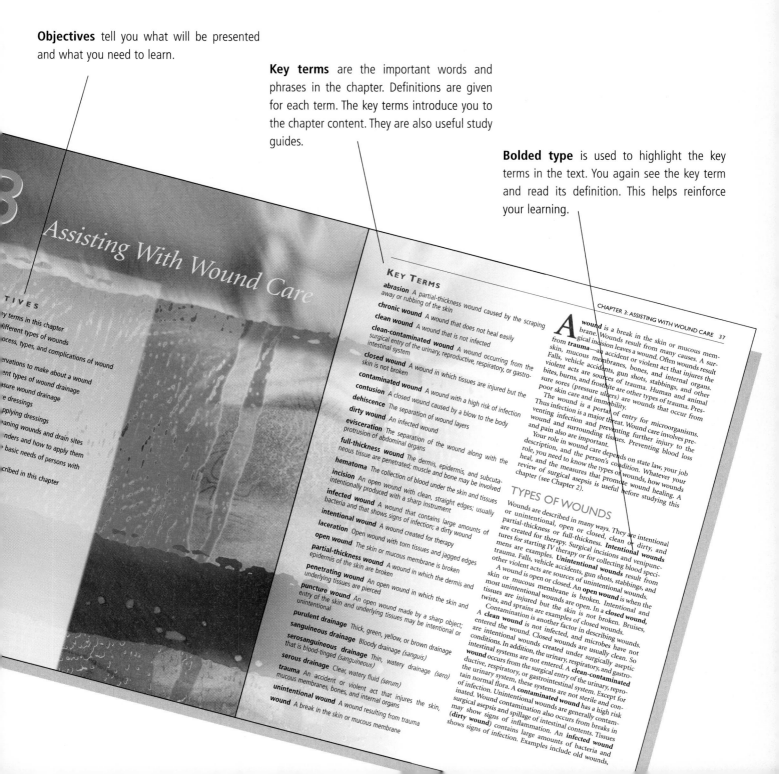

Assisting With Wound Care

OBJECTIVES

- key terms in this chapter
- different types of wounds
- process, types, and complications of wound
- observations to make about a wound
- different types of wound drainage
- measure wound drainage
- the dressings
- applying dressings
- cleaning wounds and drain sites
- binders and how to apply them
- the basic needs of persons with
- described in this chapter

KEY TERMS

abrasion A partial-thickness wound caused by the scraping away or rubbing of the skin

chronic wound A wound that does not heal easily

clean wound A wound that is not infected

clean-contaminated wound A wound occurring from the surgical entry of the urinary, reproductive, respiratory, or gastro-intestinal system

closed wound A wound in which tissues are injured but the skin is not broken

contaminated wound A wound with a high risk of infection

contusion A closed wound caused by a blow to the body

dehiscence The separation of wound layers

dirty wound An infected wound

evisceration The separation of the wound along with the protrusion of abdominal organs

full-thickness wound The dermis, epidermis, and subcutaneous tissue are penetrated; muscle and bone may be involved

hematoma The collection of blood under the skin and tissues

incision An open wound with clean, straight edges; usually intentionally produced with a sharp instrument

infected wound A wound that contains large amounts of bacteria and that shows signs of infection; a dirty wound

intentional wound A wound created for therapy

laceration Open wound with torn tissues and jagged edges

open wound The skin or mucous membrane is broken

partial-thickness wound A wound in which the dermis and epidermis of the skin are broken

penetrating wound An open wound in which the skin and underlying tissues are pierced

puncture wound An open wound made by a sharp object; entry of the skin and underlying tissues may be intentional or unintentional

purulent drainage Thick, green, yellow, or brown drainage

sanguineous drainage Bloody drainage (*sanguis*)

serosanguineous drainage Thin, watery drainage that is blood-tinged (*sero*) (*sanguineous*)

serous drainage Clear, watery fluid (*serum*)

trauma An accident or violent act that injures the skin, mucous membranes, bones, and internal organs

unintentional wound A wound resulting from trauma

wound A break in the skin or mucous membrane

A **wound** is a break in the skin or mucous membrane. Wounds result from many causes. A surgical incision leaves a wound. Often wounds result from **trauma**—an accident or violent act that injures the skin, mucous membranes, bones, and internal organs. Falls, vehicle accidents, gun shots, stabbings, and other violent acts are sources of trauma. Human and animal bites, burns, and frostbite are other types of trauma. Pressure sores (pressure ulcers) are wounds that occur from poor skin care and immobility.

The wound is a portal of entry for microorganisms. Thus infection is a major threat. Wound care involves preventing infection and preventing further injury to the wound and surrounding tissues. Preventing blood loss and pain also are important.

Your role in wound care depends on state law, your job description, and the person's condition. Whatever your role, you need to know the types of wounds, how wounds heal, and the measures that promote wound healing. A review of surgical asepsis is useful before studying this chapter (see Chapter 2).

TYPES OF WOUNDS

Wounds are described in many ways. They are intentional or unintentional, open or closed, clean or dirty, and partial-thickness or full-thickness. Surgical incisions and venipunctures for starting IV therapy or for collecting blood specimens are examples. **Unintentional wounds** result from trauma. Falls, vehicle accidents, gun shots, stabbings, and other violent acts are sources of unintentional wounds.

A wound is open or closed. An **open wound** is when the skin or mucous membrane is broken. Intentional and most unintentional wounds are open. In a **closed wound,** tissues are injured but the skin is not broken. Bruises, twists, and sprains are examples of closed wounds.

Contamination is another factor in describing wounds. A **clean wound** is not infected, and microbes have not entered the wound. Closed wounds are usually clean. So are intentional wounds created under surgically aseptic conditions. In addition, the urinary, respiratory, and intestinal systems are not entered. A **clean-contaminated wound** occurs from the surgical entry of the urinary, respiratory, or gastrointestinal system. Except for the urinary system, these systems are not sterile and contain normal flora. A **contaminated wound** has a high risk of infection. Unintentional wounds are generally contaminated. Wound contamination also occurs from breaks in surgical asepsis and spillage of intestinal contents. Tissues may show signs of inflammation. An **infected wound** (**dirty wound**) contains large amounts of bacteria and shows signs of infection. Examples include old wounds,

Focus on. . . segments highlight special considerations for children, older persons, and home care.

Boxes and tables contain important rules, principles, guidelines, signs and symptoms, and other information in a list format. They identify important information and are useful study guides for reviewing.

Color illustrations and photographs visually present a key idea, concept, or procedure step. They help you apply and remember the written material.

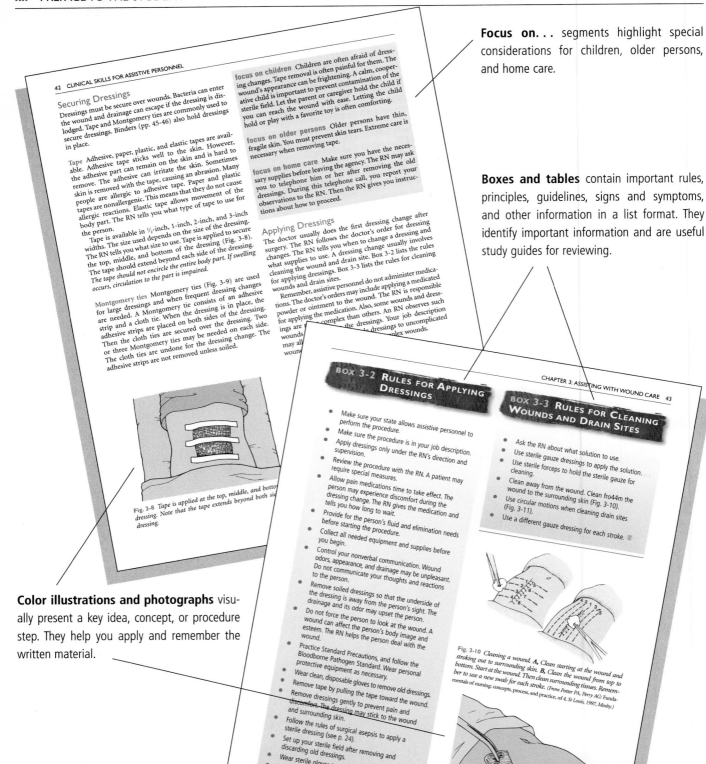

42 CLINICAL SKILLS FOR ASSISTIVE PERSONNEL

Securing Dressings

Dressings must be secure over wounds. Bacteria can enter the wound and drainage can escape if the dressing is dislodged. Tape and Montgomery ties are commonly used to secure dressings. Binders (pp. 45-46) also hold dressings in place.

Tape Adhesive, paper, plastic, and elastic tapes are available. Adhesive tape sticks well to the skin. However, the adhesive part can remain on the skin and is hard to remove. The adhesive can irritate the skin. Sometimes skin is removed with the tape, causing an abrasion. Many people are allergic to adhesive tape. Paper and plastic tapes are nonallergenic. This means that they do not cause allergic reactions. Elastic tape allows movement of the body part. The RN tells you what type of tape to use for the person.

Tape is available in ½-inch, 1-inch, 2-inch, and 3-inch widths. The size used depends on the size of the dressing. The RN tells you what size to use. Tape is applied to secure the top, middle, and bottom of the dressing (Fig. 3-8). *The tape should extend beyond each side of the dressing. If swelling occurs, circulation to the part is impaired.*

Montgomery ties Montgomery ties (Fig. 3-9) are used for large dressings and when frequent dressing changes are needed. A Montgomery tie consists of an adhesive strip and a cloth tie. When the dressing is in place, the adhesive strips are placed on both sides of the dressing. Then the cloth ties are secured over the dressing. Two or three Montgomery ties may be needed on each side. The cloth ties are undone for the dressing change. The adhesive strips are not removed unless soiled.

focus on children Children are often afraid of dressing changes. Tape removal is often painful for them. The wound's appearance can be frightening. A calm, cooperative child is important to prevent contamination of the sterile field. Let the parent or caregiver hold the child if you can reach the wound with ease. Letting the child hold or play with a favorite toy is often comforting.

focus on older persons Older persons have thin, fragile skin. You must prevent skin tears. Extreme care is necessary when removing tape.

focus on home care Make sure you have the necessary supplies before leaving the agency. The RN may ask you to telephone him or her after removing the old dressings. During this telephone call, you report your observations to the RN. Then the RN gives you instructions about how to proceed.

Applying Dressings

The doctor usually does the first dressing change after surgery. The RN follows the doctor's order for dressing changes. The RN tells you when to change a dressing and what supplies to use. A dressing change usually involves cleaning the wound and drain site. Box 3-2 lists the rules for applying dressings. Box 3-3 lists the rules for cleaning wounds and drain sites.

Remember, assistive personnel do not administer medications. The doctor's orders may include applying a medicated powder or ointment to the wound. The RN is responsible for applying the medication. Also, some wounds and dressings are [more] complex than others. An RN observes such [wounds and] the dressings. Your job description may all[ow]... dressings to uncomplicated wounds...plex wounds.

Fig. 3-8 *Tape is applied at the top, middle, and bott[om of the] dressing. Note that the tape extends beyond both si[des of the] dressing.*

CHAPTER 3: ASSISTING WITH WOUND CARE 43

BOX 3-2 RULES FOR APPLYING DRESSINGS

- Make sure your state allows assistive personnel to perform the procedure.
- Make sure the procedure is in your job description.
- Apply dressings only under the RN's direction and supervision.
- Review the procedure with the RN. A patient may require special measures.
- Allow pain medications time to take effect. The person may experience discomfort during the dressing change. The RN gives the medication and tells you how long to wait.
- Provide for the person's fluid and elimination needs before starting the procedure.
- Collect all needed equipment and supplies before you begin.
- Control your nonverbal communication. Wound odors, appearance, and drainage may be unpleasant. Do not communicate your thoughts and reactions to the person.
- Remove soiled dressings so that the underside of the dressing is away from the person's sight. The drainage and its odor may upset the person.
- Do not force the person to look at the wound. A wound can affect the person's body image and esteem. The RN helps the person deal with the wound.
- Practice Standard Precautions, and follow the Bloodborne Pathogen Standard. Wear personal protective equipment as necessary.
- Wear clean, disposable gloves to remove old dressings.
- Remove tape by pulling the tape toward the wound.
- Remove dressings gently to prevent pain and discomfort. The dressing may stick to the wound and surrounding skin.
- Follow the rules of surgical asepsis to apply a sterile dressing (see p. 24).
- Set up your sterile field after removing and discarding old dressings.
- Wear sterile gloves to apply new dressings.
- Follow the rules for cleaning wounds and drain sites (see Box 3-3). ❀

BOX 3-3 RULES FOR CLEANING WOUNDS AND DRAIN SITES

- Ask the RN about what solution to use.
- Use sterile gauze dressings to apply the solution.
- Use sterile forceps to hold the sterile gauze for cleaning.
- Clean away from the wound. Clean fro44m the wound to the surrounding skin (Fig. 3-10).
- Use circular motions when cleaning drain sites (Fig. 3-11).
- Use a different gauze dressing for each stroke. ❀

Fig. 3-10 *Cleaning a wound. A, Clean starting at the wound and stroking out to surrounding skin. B, Clean the wound from top to bottom. Start at the wound. Then clean surrounding tissues. Remember to use a new swab for each stroke. (From Potter PA, Perry AG: Fundamentals of nursing: concepts, process, and practice, ed 4, St Louis, 1997, Mosby.)*

Fig. 3-11 *Cleaning a drain site. Clean in circular motions starting at the drain site. Use a new swab for each stroke.*

Procedures are written in a step-by-step format. They are divided into pre-procedure, procedure, and post-procedure sections for easy studying.

Summaries at the end of the chapter identify important content and review what you have learned.

PRIMING IV TUBING

PRE-PROCEDURE

1 Review the procedure with the RN.
2 Wash your hands.
3 Collect the following as directed by the RN:
  • IV solution (get this from the RN if it contains medications)
  • Infusion set
  • IV pole
  • Alcohol swabs
  • Disposable gloves
  • IV gown (sleeves snap close)
  • IV label
4 Check the solution container:
  a Check to see that the solution is clear and free of particles.

  b Make sure the container is unopened.
  c Make sure the container does not leak.
  d Check the container for cracks.
  e Check the expiration date.
5 Ask the RN to check the IV solution. You must make sure that you have the right solution.
6 Arrange equipment on a clean work area.
7 Identify the patient. Check the ID bracelet with the assignment sheet.
8 Explain what you are going to do.
9 Provide for privacy.

PROCEDURE

10 Help the person tend to any personal hygiene or elimination needs. Wear gloves. Clean and return equipment to its proper place. Wash your hands.
11 Help the person change into the IV gown.
12 Write the person's name and the date and time on the IV label.
13 Apply the IV label to the container. Apply it so that it can be read after hanging the container (Fig. 7-12, p. 128).
14 Open the sterile infusion set. Make sure the protective caps are on the spike and the needle adapter.
15 Open the clamp, and move it to the end of the drip chamber.
16 Close the clamp all the way.
17 Remove the protective cap from the container (Fig. 7-13, p. 128). The opening is sterile. Do not touch the opening.
18 Clean the rubber stopper on a glass container with an alcohol swab.
19 Remove the protective cap from the spike. The spike is sterile. Do not touch the spike. Do not let anything touch the spike.

20 Insert the spike into the container (Fig. 7-14, p. 128).
21 Hang the solution container on the IV pole.
22 Squeeze the drip chamber gently. Squeeze until the drip chamber is about one-half full (Fig. 7-15, p. 128).
23 Remove the protective cap from the needle adapter. Save the cap for step 28. The adapter is sterile. Do not touch the adapter. Do not let anything touch the adapter.
24 Hold the needle end of the tubing over a sink or container.
25 Open the clamp slowly. Open it only halfway.
26 Allow fluid to flow through the tubing until it is free of air and bubbles.
27 Close the clamp.
28 Put the protective cap on the needle adapter. Do not touch the adapter.
29 Check the tube for bubbles. Gently tap tubing at a bubble site to remove the bubble (Fig. 7-16, p. 128).

POST-PROCEDURE

30 Make sure the person is comfortable.
31 Make sure the call bell is within reach.
32 Raise or lower bed rails as instructed by the RN.
33 Tell the patient that the RN will start the IV.

34 Unscreen the person.
35 Tell the RN that the tubing is primed. Report any patient observations.
36 Wash your hands.

CH

SUMMARY

Blood transfusions can save a person's life. They can also kill if the wrong blood is given to the wrong person. Therefore blood administration requires the knowledge, skills, and judgment of RNs. Your state and job description may allow you to assist the RN.

REVIEW QUESTIONS

Circle the best answer.

1 Which carry oxygen to the cells?
  a Antibodies
  b Antigens
  c Hemoglobin
  d Platelets

2 The liquid portion of blood is called
  a Plasma
  b Erythrocytes
  c Hemoglobin
  d Hemolysis

3 Which is necessary for blood clotting?
  a Plasma
  b Erythroctyes
  c Hemoglobin
  d Platelets

4 A person's blood has the type B antigen. The person's blood type is
  a Type A
  b Type B
  c Type AB
  d Type O

5 A person with type O blood
  a Has the type A and type B antigens
  b Is Rh+
  c Has no antigens
  d Is Rh−

6 Who can receive type O blood?
  a Persons with type A blood or type B blood
  b Persons with type AB blood

  c Persons with type
  d All of the above

7 You are asked to obtain blood from the b... The following are checked with the laboratory technician *except*
  a The person's blood type
  b The person's Rh factor
  c The person's ID bracelet
  d The blood's expiration date

8 The most critical time for a transfusion reaction is
  a The first 15 minutes of the infusion
  b The first hour of the infusion
  c The last hour of the infusion
  d The first hour after the infusion

9 A patient is receiving a blood transfusion. The person complains of a backache and chills. What should you do?
  a Measure the person's vital signs.
  b Tell the RN immediately.
  c Stop the transfusion.
  d Ask about other signs and symptoms.

10 The following are signs and symptoms of a transfusion reaction *except*
  a Wound drainage
  b Hypotension
  c Tachycardia
  d Chest pain

Answers to these questions are on p. 179

Review questions are a useful study guide. They help you to review what you have learned. They can also be used when studying for a test or the competency evaluation. Answers are given at the back of the book on page 179.

Contents

Clinical Skills for
Assistive Personnel

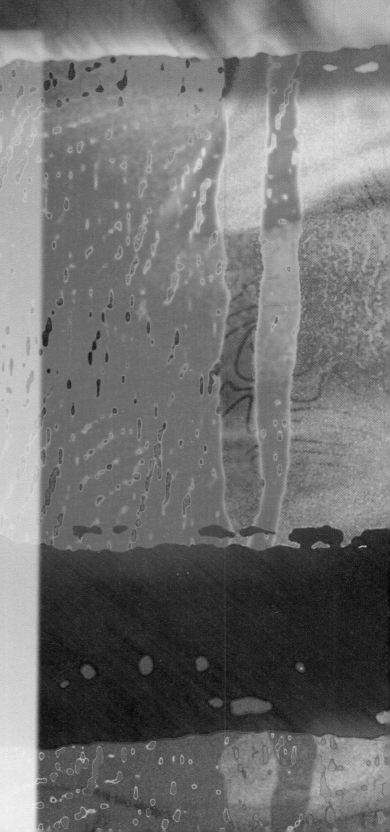

Assistive Personnel

OBJECTIVES

- Define the key terms in this chapter
- Explain the history and current trends affecting assistive personnel
- Describe nurse practice acts and their purposes
- Explain how nurse practice acts affect assistive personnel
- Describe how the Omnibus Budget Reconciliation Act of 1987 affects assistive personnel
- Explain the functions, roles, and responsibilities of assistive personnel
- Describe the educational requirements for assistive personnel
- Describe the delegation process and the "five rights of delegation"
- Explain how you should use the "five rights of delegation"
- Explain your responsibilities when you accept a delegated task
- Describe what you should do when you need to refuse a delegated task
- Describe how you can work well with the nursing and health care teams
- Describe ethical behavior on the job
- Explain what is meant by harassment and sexual harassment

KEY TERMS

accountable Being responsible for one's actions and the actions of others who perform delegated tasks; answering questions about and explaining one's actions and the actions of others

confidentiality Trusting others with personal and private information

courtesy A polite, considerate, or helpful comment or act

delegate Authorizing another person to perform a task

gossip Spreading rumors or talking about the private matters of others

harassment Troubling, tormenting, offending, or worrying a person by one's behavior or comments

preceptor A teacher

responsibility The duty or obligation to perform some act or function

task A function, procedure, activity, or work that does not require professional knowledge or judgment

work ethics Behavior in the workplace

Assistive personnel assist nurses in providing patient care. Some of the many different titles for assistive personnel are listed in Box 1-1. Supervised by RNs, assistive personnel perform selected nursing tasks. State laws, job descriptions, the patient's condition, and the amount of supervision needed and available influence what assistive personnel can do.

HISTORY

Nursing practice has a long history involving assistive personnel. For decades, they have assisted nurses in giving patient care. Commonly called *nurse's aides* or *nursing assistants,* assistive personnel gave basic bedside nursing care. Bathing and feeding patients were common tasks, along with making beds, repositioning, and assisting with elimination. Their work was essentially the same in hospitals and nursing homes throughout the United States. Until the 1980s, no training or experience was required. On-the-job training was given by the RNs. Some hospitals, nursing homes, and schools offered nursing assistant courses.

Before the 1980s, team nursing was the common nursing care pattern. Team members included RNs, LPNs/LVNs, and nursing assistants. An RN was the team leader.

BOX 1-1 TITLES FOR ASSISTIVE PERSONNEL

- Certified Nursing Assistant
- Clinical Technician
- Health Care Assistant
- Health Care Technician
- Licensed Nursing Assistant
- Nurse's Aide
- Nurse Extender
- Nurse Technician
- Nursing Support Technician
- Patient Care Assistant
- Patient Care Attendant
- Patient Care Monitor
- Patient Care Technician
- Patient Care Worker
- Support Partner ✻

The RN made team member assignments according to each patient's needs and condition. The education and experiences of each staff member also influenced assignments. Team members communicated with the team leader about patient care and observations.

Primary nursing became popular in the 1980s. RNs planned and gave patient care. With this nursing care pattern, hospitals eliminated many LPN/LVN and nursing assistant positions. Often only RNs were hired to give patient care.

Meanwhile, nursing homes continued to rely heavily on nursing assistants for resident care. In an effort to improve the quality of life of nursing home residents, the U.S. Congress passed the Omnibus Budget Reconciliation Act (OBRA) of 1987. The law sets minimum training and competency evaluation requirements for nursing assistants working in nursing homes. This law requires each state to set rules for nursing assistant training and evaluation. A state's requirements must be met before a person can work as a nursing assistant in a nursing home in that state.

Home care also increased during the 1980s. Prospective payment systems greatly impacted this trend. Prospective payment systems limit how much insurance companies, Medicare, and Medicaid pay for health care. Prospective relates to *before* care. The cost of treating an illness and the length of hospital stay are predetermined. If the costs are less than the predetermined amount, the hospital keeps the extra money. If the costs are more, the hospital takes the loss. In addition, the person can stay in the hospital only a certain length of time. The longer the person stays, the greater the loss to the hospital. Therefore patients are discharged earlier than in the past. These persons are often still quite ill. Home care may be required.

focus on home care To help ensure quality home care, many states have training and competency requirements for persons employed to give home care. These persons are called *home health care assistants* or *home health aides*. If a home care agency receives Medicare funds, assistive personnel must meet federal training and competency evaluation requirements. As it is for long-term care, 75 hours of training is required.

CURRENT TRENDS

The continued rising costs of health care became a major issue in the early 1990s. The goal was to control and reduce these costs and to provide all persons with access to health care. Insurance companies, Medicare, and Medicaid further reduced payments for treating specific illnesses. Meanwhile, health care costs continued to increase.

Efforts to reduce health care costs included:

- *Hospital closings*—Many hospitals closed for financial reasons. The amount of money coming into the hospital was not enough to meet the hospital's expenses.

- *Hospital mergers*—Hospitals merged to share resources and to avoid offering the same costly services. For example, instead of two hospitals offering cardiac surgery services, only one does. The other hospital may offer maternity and pediatric services.

- *Health care systems*—Health care agencies join together as one provider of care (Fig. 1-1). The system may include hospitals, nursing homes, home care agencies, ambulance services, hospice settings, and doctors. Medical supply stores are also common for home care. The system may serve a community or a large geographic area. Patients use the system's services. For example, a hospital patient needs long-term care. The system's ambulance service is used to transfer the person from the hospital to the system-owned nursing home. When the person is ready for discharge from the nursing home, home care is arranged with the system's home care agency. The person's care is kept within the system, maximizing the system's resources.

- *Managed care*—Many insurance companies have contracts with doctors, hospitals, and health care systems. The contracts provide for reduced rates or discounts. The insured person uses those doctors and facilities offering the lower rates. If others are used, the care is covered in part or not at all. Costs not covered by insurance must be paid by the patient. Health maintenance organizations (HMOs) and preferred provider organizations (PPOs) are common managed care arrangements (Box 1-2).

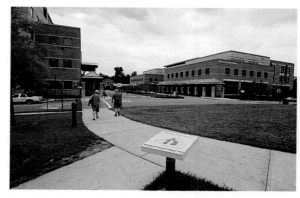

Fig. 1-1 *The hospital and doctors' offices are part of a health care system. (Courtesy Anne Arundel Health System, Inc., Annapolis, Md.)*

- *Return to a nursing staff mix*—Instead of hiring only RNs, hospitals began hiring assistive personnel. The titles listed in Box 1-1 and others emerged as assistive personnel assumed the nursing assistant role and were assigned complex nursing tasks. Today more and more hospitals are hiring assistive personnel. Some hospitals provide a training program for assistive personnel. Others require completion of a state-approved nursing assistant training and competency evaluation program for employment. Additional training is given for those nursing tasks not included in the training program but that are part of the person's job description.

- *Patient-focused care and cross-training*—This moves hospital services from departments to the bedside. Staff members are cross-trained to perform basic skills provided by other health team members. Nurses and assistive personnel are often cross-trained to collect blood specimens (phlebotomy) and take electrocardiograms (ECGs, EKGs). For example, a doctor orders a blood test for Ms. Tyler. The nurse tells the unit secretary, who then calls the laboratory. The laboratory secretary tells a medical laboratory technician. The technician sends a staff member to Ms. Tyler's room to draw the blood sample. Five people are involved so far. With patient-focused care and

cross-training, Ms. Tyler's blood is drawn when the order is given. She does not wait for laboratory staff to be notified and arrive. She is served faster and with less staff. Staff members are used in efficient and productive ways. The number of people caring for each patient is also reduced.

STATE AND FEDERAL LAWS

The tasks performed by assistive personnel vary from state to state and facility to facility. Often variation occurs within facilities. For example, assistive personnel in the emergency room, medical-surgical units, and intensive care units may be trained to perform different tasks.

Unlike nursing assistant training and practice in nursing home settings, the work of assistive personnel in hospitals is currently not well-defined. Concerns about the training and job descriptions of assistive personnel are prompting many states to study the issue. Many states are attempting to control and regulate the training and practice of assistive personnel working in hospitals. State nurse practice acts and OBRA provide some direction.

Nurse Practice Acts

Each state has a nurse practice act. Intended to protect public welfare and safety, the law regulates nursing practice in that state. Definitions are given for RNs and LPNs/LVNs, and the scope of their practice is described. The law provides for RN and LPN education and licensing requirements. The law protects the public from persons practicing nursing without a license. That is, it prevents persons who do not meet the state's education and licensing requirements from performing nursing functions.

In addition, the law allows for revoking or suspending a nurse's license to practice. The reasons for such disciplinary action include:

- Being convicted of a crime in any state
- Selling or distributing drugs
- Using the patient's drugs for oneself
- Endangering patient safety from the excessive use of alcohol or drugs
- Demonstrating grossly negligent nursing practice
- Being convicted of child abuse or neglect
- Violating the provisions of the act and its rules and regulations
- Demonstrating incompetent behaviors
- Aiding or assisting another person to violate the act and its rules and regulations
- Making medical diagnoses or prescribing medicines and treatments

BOX 1-2 TYPES OF MANAGED CARE

Health Maintenance Organization (HMO)—provides health care services for a prepaid fee. For the fee, persons receive all needed services offered by the organization. Some need only an annual physical examination, but others require hospital care. Whatever services are used, the cost is covered by the prepaid fee. HMOs emphasize preventing disease and maintaining health. Keeping someone healthy costs far less than treating illness.

Preferred Provider Organization (PPO)—is a group of doctors and hospitals that provides health care at reduced rates. Usually the arrangement is made between the PPO and an employer or an insurance company. Employees or those insured are given reduced rates for the services used. The person can choose any doctor or hospital in the PPO. ✳

Because a state's nurse practice act defines nursing and its scope of practice, it is used to determine the nursing tasks that assistive personnel can perform. Legal and advisory opinions about assistive personnel are based on the act. So are any state laws that regulate assistive personnel. If you perform a task beyond the legal limits of your role, you could be practicing nursing without a license. This creates serious legal problems for you and the RN supervising your work.

The Omnibus Budget Reconciliation Act of 1987

In 1987 the U.S. Congress passed the Omnibus Budget Reconciliation Act (OBRA). This law applies to all 50 states. The law addresses training for nursing assistants working in long-term care. It requires each state to have a nursing assistant training and competency evaluation program. Assistive personnel working in nursing homes and hospital long-term care units must meet federal and state training and competency requirements.

State requirements vary. However, OBRA requires at least 75 hours of instruction. Sixteen of those hours involve supervised practical training. Such training occurs in a laboratory or clinical setting. The student actually performs nursing care and procedures on another person. This practical training (clinical practicum or clinical experience) is supervised by an RN.

The training program includes the knowledge and skills needed by nursing assistants to give basic nursing care. Areas of study include:

- Communication
- Infection control
- Safety and emergency procedures
- Residents' rights
- Basic nursing skills
- Personal care skills
- Feeding techniques
- Elimination procedures
- Skin care
- Transferring, positioning, and turning techniques
- Dressing
- Ambulating residents
- Range-of-motion exercises

The competency evaluation program includes a written test and a skills test. The number of test questions on the *written test* varies from state to state. The *skills* evaluation involves demonstrating nursing skills learned in the training program.

OBRA requires that each state have a nursing assistant registry. The registry is an official record or listing of persons who have successfully completed a state-approved nursing assistant training and competency evaluation program. Information about a nursing assistant abusing or neglecting a resident is part of the registry information. So are findings about the dishonest use of property.

ROLES, FUNCTIONS, AND RESPONSIBILITIES

Nurse practice acts, OBRA, state laws, and legal and advisory opinions give direction for the roles, functions, and responsibilities of assistive personnel. To protect patients from harm, you must understand what you can do, what you cannot do, and the legal limits of your role.

Assistive personnel function under the supervision of RNs. You assist RNs and LPNs/LVNs in giving care. You also perform nursing procedures and tasks involved in the person's care. Often you function without an RN in the room. At other times you help nurses give bedside nursing care. In some facilities you assist doctors with diagnostic procedures. The rules listed in Box 1-3 should help you understand your role.

Assistive personnel functions and responsibilities vary among states and facilities. The procedures in this textbook are performed by assistive personnel. Some are more complex and advanced than others. Before you perform a nursing task:

BOX 1-3 RULES FOR ASSISTIVE PERSONNEL

- You are an assistant to the RN.
- An RN determines and supervises your work.
- You do not decide what should or should not be done for a person.
- If you do not understand directions or instructions, ask the RN for clarification before going to the person.
- Perform no task that you have not been prepared to do or that you do not feel comfortable performing without an RN's supervision.
- Perform only those tasks that are allowed by your state and that are in your job description. ✳

- Your state must allow assistive personnel to perform the task
- The task must be part of your job description
- You must have the necessary education and training
- You must have the necessary supervision

Generally, you assist an RN in meeting a person's hygiene, safety, nutrition, exercise, elimination, and oxygen needs. Related functions include lifting and moving patients, observing them, helping promote physical comfort, and collecting specimens. You also assist with patient admissions and discharges and measure temperatures, pulses, respirations, and blood pressures. Assistive personnel sometimes perform sterile procedures such as urinary catheterizations, dressing changes, and collection of blood specimens. Obtaining electrocardiograms is a common task for assistive personnel (Fig. 1-2).

Box 1-4 describes the limits of your role. These are the procedures and tasks that assistive personnel never perform. As stated previously, you must understand what you *cannot* do.

You must remember that state laws and legal and advisory opinions differ. Therefore you must know what assistive personnel can do in the state in which you are working. For example, if you live in Utah and move to New Hampshire, you must become familiar with the laws and rules in New Hampshire. Sometimes assistive personnel

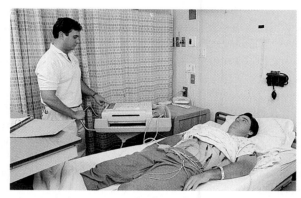

Fig. 1-2 *Assistive personnel often obtain electrocardiograms.*

BOX 1-4 ROLE LIMITS FOR ASSISTIVE PERSONNEL

- **Never give medications.** This includes medications given orally, rectally, by injection, by application to the skin, or directly into the bloodstream through an intravenous line. Giving medications is a responsibility of licensed nurses. This responsibility cannot be delegated to assistive personnel unless allowed by state law. Some states allow for the education and use of medication technicians or aides.

- **Never insert tubes or objects into body openings or remove them from the body unless allowed by your state and job description.** For example, some states allow assistive personnel to insert catheters (tubes) into the urinary bladder. Other states do not.

- **Never take oral or telephone orders from physicians.** Politely give your name and title, ask the doctor to wait, and promptly find an RN to speak with the doctor.

- **Never tell the patient or family the person's diagnosis or medical or surgical treatment plans.** The doctor is responsible for informing the person and family about the diagnosis and treatment. RNs may further clarify what the doctor said.

- **Never diagnose or prescribe treatments or medications for anyone.** Only doctors can diagnose and prescribe.

- **Never supervise other assistive personnel.** RNs are legally responsible for supervising the work of assistive personnel. You will not be trained or paid to supervise the work of others. Supervising other assistive personnel has serious legal consequences.

- **Never ignore an order or request to do something that you cannot do or that is beyond the legal limits for assistive personnel.** Promptly explain to the RN why you cannot carry out the order or request. The RN assumes you are doing what you were told to do unless you explain otherwise. Patient care cannot be neglected. ✳

work in two states. For example, you work part-time at a hospital in Illinois and part-time at another hospital in Iowa. What you are allowed to do in Illinois may be different from what you do in Iowa. You must know the laws and rules of each state.

Some assistive personnel are also emergency medical technicians (EMTs). EMTs are trained to give emergency care in settings outside of hospitals and other health care facilities. These settings are called "in the field." They work under the direction of doctors in hospital emergency rooms. Each state has laws and rules that apply to EMTs. These laws and rules are different from those for assistive personnel. What EMTs do "in the field" is very different from the work of assistive personnel. For example, Joan Woods is an EMT for a fire department. When off duty, she works as a patient care assistant at St. John's Hospital. Her state allows EMTs to start intravenous infusions (IVs) in the field. However, assistive personnel do not start IVs. Despite knowing how to start an IV, Joan cannot start IVs when working at the hospital as a patient care assistant.

The situation is similar for persons who served as medics or corpsmen in military service. For example, a medic or corpsman may be allowed to suture wounds. Assistive personnel cannot do so. When employed as assistive personnel, medics and corpsmen must follow the state laws and rules that apply to assistive personnel in that state. As with EMTs, the ability to perform a procedure or task does not give a person the right to perform that procedure or task in all settings.

The functions of assistive personnel are limited by state laws and rules. Job descriptions for assistive personnel reflect those laws and rules.

Job Description

A job description lists the responsibilities and functions you are expected to perform (Box 1-5). Always request a written job description when you apply for a job. Ask questions about the job description during your job interview. Before accepting a job, tell the employer about any functions you do not know how to do. Also advise the employer of functions you are opposed to doing for moral or religious reasons. Have a clear understanding of what is expected of you before taking a job. Do not take a job that requires you to:

- Function beyond your educational limits
- Perform acts that are against your moral or religious principles
- Act beyond the legal limits of your role
- Perform procedures and tasks that your state does not allow assistive personnel to perform

No one can force you to perform a function, task, or procedure that is beyond the legal limits of assistive personnel. That is why you must understand the roles and responsibilities of assistive personnel in your state. You also need to know the functions you can safely perform, the things you should never do, and your job description.

EDUCATIONAL REQUIREMENTS

Each agency has its own educational requirements for assistive personnel. These requirements are based on state laws or recommendations that limit the functions, roles, and responsibilities of assistive personnel. Your training may be in a community college, technical school, hospital, or nursing home.

When employed, you will complete the facility's orientation program. The facility's policies and procedures are explained, and your skills are checked. That is, the facility has you perform nursing procedures and tasks to make sure you can do them safely and correctly. Also, you are shown how to use the facility's supplies and equipment.

Some facilities have clinical preceptor programs. A **preceptor** is a teacher. In a clinical preceptor program, RNs are trained to teach and train assistive personnel in the clinical area (Fig. 1-3). For example, you complete a training program for assistive personnel. You are going to work with pediatric patients. You are assigned to an RN preceptor who works with you and supervises your work for a period of time. The RN helps you adjust to your role, shows you how to use the facility's equipment and supplies, answers your questions, and makes sure that you give safe care. Depending on the agency, the preceptor program can last from 6 weeks to 3 months. It is designed to help you succeed in your new role and to ensure quality and safe patient care.

Text continued on p. 10

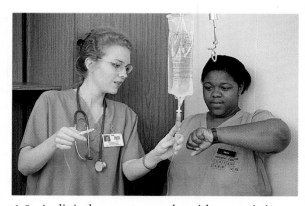

Fig. 1-3 *A clinical preceptor works with an assistive person.*

BOX 1-5 JOB DESCRIPTION FOR ASSISTIVE PERSONNEL

OSF SAINT FRANCIS MEDICAL CENTER
PEORIA, ILLINOIS
JOB DESCRIPTION

JOB TITLE: Patient Care Tech

DEPARTMENT: Various Services

DIVISION: Patient Services

GENERAL SUMMARY:

Reporting to the Patient Care Manager and according to department standards, functions as a member of the Patient Care Team to provide appropriate basic care to patients based on the ages of the patients served on the unit. This includes taking vital signs, assisting patients with activities of daily living, blood draws, dressing changes, foley catheterizations, EKGs, and observing patients for physical/emotional changes. Records pertinent information in patient charts and communicates with other patient care team members to ensure continuity of care. The following are general characteristics of this job, although duties may vary by assigned shift.

CORPORATE PHILOSOPHY:

It is the obligation of each employee of OSF Saint Francis Medical Center to abide by and promote the Corporate Philosophy, Values, Mission, and Vision of The Sisters of the Third Order of St. Francis.

PRINCIPAL DUTIES AND RESPONSIBILITIES: (The following duties and responsibilities are all essential job functions, as defined by the ADA, except for those that begin with the word "May.")

1. Takes and records patients' vital signs including temperature, pulse, BP, weight, respiration as prescribed by nursing protocol or physician order.

2. Assists patients with activities of daily living including personal hygiene and grooming, bathing, eating, back rubs, etc. Provides patients with bedpans or urinals, empties and cleans, or assist patients to commode or bathroom.

3. Performs various technical nursing procedures according to protocol, including: maintaining oxygen equipment, performing oral and nasopharyngeal suctioning, routine incisional care, performing urinary bladder catheterization, giving tube feedings, changing sterile dressings, providing skin care, sitz baths, enemas, applying and changing nonsterile dressings and pads, applying warm and cold compresses, ointments, etc. Records activities in patient records.

4. Monitors, measures, and records patients' intake and output according to established nursing protocol and physician orders.

5. Observes patients (physical appearance, attitude) and communicates any changes or pertinent information related to the patient's health to appropriate team members.

6. Assists patients with ambulating or exercising. Ensures patient safety by following established safety standards. Repositions patients in chairs and beds.

7. Delivers patient meals and nourishments. In doing so, feeds or assists patients that require assistance in feeding and documents portion of meal completed. Collects meal trays at end of meal and assists with menu marking as needed, including appropriate substitutions and initiates snacks according to patient needs.

Modified from OSF Saint Francis Medical Center, Peoria, Illinois.

Continued

BOX 1-5 JOB DESCRIPTION FOR ASSISTIVE PERSONNEL—CONT'D

PRINCIPAL DUTIES AND RESPONSIBILITIES—cont'd:

8. Collects patient specimens (e.g., urine, stool, sputum, blood), labels, and sends to laboratory for analysis, and communicates to appropriate team member.

9. Completes EKGs per physician orders. In doing so, attaches electrode leads to various parts of the patients arms and chests. Conducts the EKG and records the heart rhythms. Monitors patients during test to ensure patients are relaxed and remain still in effort to reduce artifacts. Monitors rhythms for abnormal patterns and notifies appropriate patient care team members of critical heart irregularities. Keys information into EKG machine to note position of electrodes and/or manually marks rhythms strips.

10. Obtains blood specimens from patients per physician's order. Applies tourniquet to arm, locates accessible vein, swabs puncture site with anticeptic, and inserts needle into vein to draw blood into collection tube. May prick finger to draw blood, depending on type of specimen test required/requested.

11. As a member of the patient care team, provides support to other patient care team members by assisting in patient care and clerical functions including, but not limited to:

    • Responding to patients' call lights. In doing so, identifies patient needs and provides patient with appropriate response or communicates needs to appropriate team member
    • Passing water, assisting patients when dressing, etc.
    • Providing patients with blankets, pillows, and additional linen when needed
    • Collecting trash, red bagging as needed
    • Assisting in transporting patients to various departments as needed
    • Providing directions to patients/visitors

12. Transfers patients from beds onto gurneys or into wheelchairs (with assistance of other patient care team members when required). Ensures patients' safety by following proper lifting and patient transferring techniques.

13. Keeps patient rooms neat, clean, and orderly. Changes patients' bed linens on a regularly scheduled basis or as needed. Cleans unit's ancillary rooms upon request.

14. Ensures patient and supply rooms are properly stocked with necessities including clean linen, ice water, etc.

15. Attends mandatory department of Medical Center meetings, inservices, and appropriate work-related educational programs.

16. Develops and maintains a positive working relationship with team members, department and Medical Center personnel, and patients/visitors.

17. Supports and is involved in the Medical Center's continuous quality improvement efforts designed to increase patient outcomes, increase patient satisfaction, and improve the utilization of the Medical Center's human, capital, and physical resources.

KNOWLEDGE, SKILLS, AND ABILITIES REQUIRED:

1. The job incumbent is required to demonstrate the knowledge and skills necessary to provide patient care appropriate to the age of the patients served on the unit. This requires that the incumbent demonstrate knowledge of the principles of growth and development as well as the physical, emotional and psycho-social needs of the patient population served.

2. Work requires ability to read, write, and communicate effectively at a level generally acquired through completion of a high school education. Must be 17 years old to be considered for position.

BOX 1-5 JOB DESCRIPTION FOR ASSISTIVE PERSONNEL—CONT'D

KNOWLEDGE, SKILLS, AND ABILITIES REQUIRED—cont'd:

3. Work requires 3 to 4 months of unit-specific orientation and on-the-job training to become familiar with work routines and location of equipment and supplies and to develop proficiencies in patient care tech duties.

4. Work requires the interpersonal skills necessary to comfort patients, family members, and/or significant others; and to communicate effectively with other patient care providers.

5. Work requires analytical ability necessary to prioritize work load.

PHYSICAL REQUIREMENTS: (The following statements describe the physical abilities required to perform the essential job functions, although exceptions may be made to these requirements based on the principle of reasonable accommodation.)

1. Work requires the ability to lift objects weighing up to 60 pounds on a daily basis.

2. Work requires ability to carry objects weighing up to 20 pounds on a daily basis.

3. Work requires ability to stand for 3 or more hours at a time.

4. Work requires ability to stoop and bend, ability to reach and grab with arms and hands, manual dexterity, ability to communicate with others, and color vision.

5. Work requires ability to push and/or pull wheelchairs, gurneys, beds, or supply carts on a hourly basis.

6. Work requires ability to lift and position patients on a hourly basis.

REPORTING RELATIONSHIPS:

1. Reports to the Patient Care Manager.

2. Functions as a member of a self-directed work team. In doing so, provides support to patient care team members by assisting in patient care duties and clerical functions as needed.

WORKING CONDITIONS:

1. Works on a patient care unit where there is exposure to infectious disease, although potential for personal harm or bodily injury is limited when employee follows all safety procedures and uses appropriate safety equipment.

2. Work requires the performance of various unpleasant patient care tasks on a daily basis.

The above is intended to describe the general content of and requirements for the performance of this job. It is not to be construed as an exhaustive statement of duties, responsibilities, or requirements. ✳

DELEGATION

Nurse practice acts give RNs and LPNs/LVNs certain responsibilities and the authority to perform nursing tasks. A **responsibility** is the duty or obligation to perform some act or function. For example, RNs are responsible for the nursing process and for nursing care. They also supervise LPNs/LVNs and assistive personnel. Only RNs can carry out these responsibilities. They cannot give these responsibilities to other nursing team members.

In nursing, a **task** is a function, procedure, activity, or work that does not require professional knowledge or judgment. **Delegate** means authorizing another person to perform a task. However, the person must be competent to perform the task in a given situation. Determining competency is part of the delegation process.

Who Can Delegate

Nurse practice acts allow RNs to delegate tasks to LPNs/LVNs and assistive personnel. Some states allow LPNs/LVNs to delegate tasks to assistive personnel.

When making delegation decisions, nurses must protect the patient's health and safety. The delegating nurse remains accountable for the delegated task. To be **accountable** means to be responsible for one's actions and the actions of others who perform delegated tasks. It also involves answering questions about and explaining one's actions and the actions of others.

The delegating nurse must make sure that the task is completed safely and correctly. If the RN delegates, the RN is responsible for the delegated task. If the LPN/LVN delegates, the LPN/LVN is responsible for the task. Remember, the RN is also responsible for supervising the practice of LPNs/LVNs. Therefore the RN also is accountable for the tasks that LPNs/LVNs delegate to assistive personnel. The RN is accountable for all patient care.

Assistive personnel cannot delegate. You cannot delegate any task to other assistive personnel. You can ask another assistive person to help you. However, you cannot ask or tell another person to do your work.

focus on older persons Some states allow LPNs/LVNs to have supervisory roles in long-term care settings. The LPN/LVN delegates tasks to assistive personnel. The LPN/LVN follows the delegation process and the "five rights of delegation" (see p. 11).

Delegation Process

Delegated tasks must be within the legal limits of what assistive personnel can do. Before delegating tasks to you, the RN must know:

- What tasks your state allows assistive personnel to perform

- The tasks included in your job description

- What you were taught in your training program

- What skills you learned and how they were evaluated

- About your work experiences

The RN uses this information to make delegation decisions. The RN is likely to discuss this information with you. This is so the RN can get to know you, your capabilities, and your concerns. Whenever you work with a new RN, you should meet to discuss your training and work experience. You may be a new employee or new to the nursing unit. Or the RN may be someone new. In any case, it is wise for the RN to get to know you and for you to get to know the RN.

Facility policies, guidelines, and the job description for assistive personnel state what tasks RNs can delegate to assistive personnel. These documents must be consistent with state laws and rules and legal opinions about the role of assistive personnel. However, even if a task is in your job description, an RN does not have to delegate it to you. The RN must consider the circumstances when delegating.

The RN makes delegation decisions after considering the questions in Box 1-6. The patient's needs, the task, and the person performing the task must fit. The RN can decide to delegate the task to you. Or the RN can decide not to delegate the task. If the patient's needs and the task require the knowledge, judgment, and skill of an RN, the RN completes the task. You may be asked to assist.

For example, you know how to give a complete bed bath. However, Mr. Jones has multiple injuries from an auto accident. He has neck injuries and is at risk for paralysis. His left leg is fractured in three places, and he has a full leg cast. His right lung was punctured, and he has chest tubes. He has two IVs, a retention catheter, a nasogastric tube, and a tracheostomy. In this situation, giving a bed bath to Mr. Jones is complicated. The RN gives the bath and asks you to assist.

You must not be offended or get angry if you are not allowed to perform a task that is part of your job description and that is usually delegated to you. The RN makes a decision that is best for the patient at the time. That decision also is the best for you at that time. You do not want to perform a task that requires an RN's judgment and critical thinking skills. For example, you cared for Mrs. Mills while she was in the hospital. You gave personal care, assisted with ambulation, and gave wound care. After discharge, she stayed with her son. A week later she was admitted to the hospital again. She had a right hip fracture and bruises on her face and arms. She reported falling down the stairs. The RN suspects abuse. Instead of asking you to bathe Mrs. Mills, the RN does so. The RN

BOX 1-6 FACTORS AFFECTING DELEGATION DECISIONS

- What is the patient's condition? Is it stable or likely to change?
- What are the patient's basic needs at this time?
- What is the patient's mental function at this time?
- What are the patient's emotional and spiritual needs at this time?
- Can the patient assist with his or her care? Does the patient depend on others for care?
- Is the task something the nurse can delegate?
- For this patient, does the task require the knowledge, judgment, and skill of an RN or LPN/LVN?
- How often will the RN have to assess the patient?
- Can the task harm the patient? If yes, how?
- What effect will the task have on the patient?

- Is it safe for the patient if the task is delegated to you?
- Do you have the training and experience to perform the task, given the patient's current status? Is your training documented? How were your training and skills evaluated?
- How often have you performed the task?
- What other tasks were delegated to you?
- Do you have the time to perform the task safely?
- Is an RN available to supervise you?
- How much supervision will you need?
- Will you need more directions as you perform the task?
- Is an RN available to help or take over if the patient's condition changes or problems arise? ✳

---

wants to assess Mrs. Mills for other signs of abuse and to talk with her. Although you are able to give Mrs. Mills a bath, at this time she needs the RN's assessment, judgment, and critical thinking skills.

The patient's circumstances are central factors in making delegation decisions. Delegation decisions should always result in the best care for the patient. An RN places a patient's health and safety at risk with poor delegation decisions. Also, the RN may face serious legal problems. If you perform a task that places the patient at risk, you can also face serious legal problems.

The five rights of delegation The following five rights of delegation summarize the delegation process. These are based on guidelines developed by the National Council of State Boards of Nursing, Inc.:

- *The right task*—Can the task be delegated? Does the state's nurse practice act allow the RN or LPN/LVN to delegate the task? Is the task in the job description for assistive personnel?

- *The right circumstances*—What are the patient's physical, mental, emotional, and spiritual needs at this time?

- *The right person*—Do you have the training and experience to safely perform the task for this patient?

- *The right directions and communication*—The RN must give clear directions. The RN tells you what to do, when to do it, what observations to make, and when to report back. The RN allows questions and helps you set priorities.

- *The right supervision*—The RN guides, directs, and evaluates the care you give. The RN demonstrates tasks as necessary and is available to answer questions. The less experience you have performing a task, the more supervision you need. Complex tasks require greater supervision than basic tasks. Also, the patient's circumstances affect how much supervision you need. The RN assesses how the task affected the patient and how well you performed the task. To help you learn and give better care, the RN tells you what you did well and what you can do to improve your work.

Your Role in Delegation

You must remember that you perform delegated tasks for or on a person. You must perform the task safely to protect the person from harm.

You have two choices when an RN delegates a task to you. You either *agree* or *refuse* to do the task. You should use the "five rights of delegation" to make your choice. Before accepting a delegated task, you need to answer the questions in Box 1-7 on p. 12.

BOX 1-7 THE FIVE RIGHTS OF DELEGATION FOR ASSISTIVE PERSONNEL

The right task
- Does your state allow assistive personnel to perform the task?
- Were you trained to do the task?
- Do you have experience performing the task?
- Is the task in your job description?

The right circumstances
- Do you have experience performing the task given the patient's condition and needs?
- Do you understand the purpose of the task for the patient?
- Can you perform the task safely under the current circumstances?
- Do you have the equipment and supplies to safely complete the task?

- Do you know how to use the equipment and supplies?

The right person
- Are you comfortable performing the task?
- Do you have concerns about performing the task?

The right directions and communication
- Did the RN give clear directions and instructions?
- Did you review the task with the RN?
- Do you understand what the RN expects?

The right supervision
- Is an RN available to answer questions?
- Is an RN available if the patient's condition changes or if problems occur? ✳

Modified from the National Council of State Boards of Nursing, Inc.

Accepting a task When you agree to perform a task, you are responsible for your own actions. Remember, what you do or fail to do can bring harm to the patient. *You must complete the task safely.* You must ask for help when you are unsure or have questions about a task. You must communicate with the RN by reporting what you did and your observations.

Refusing a task You have the right to say "no." Sometimes refusing to follow the RN's directions is your right and duty. You should refuse to perform a task when:

- The task is beyond the legal limits of your role
- The task is not in your job description
- You were not prepared to perform the task safely
- The task could harm the patient
- The patient's condition has changed
- You do not know how to use the supplies or equipment
- The RN's directions are unethical, illegal, or against facility policies
- The RN's directions are unclear or incomplete
- An RN is not available for supervision

Protect patients and yourself by using common sense. Ask yourself if what you are doing is safe for the person.

As explained in Box 1-4, you must never ignore an order or request to do something. You must communicate your concerns to the RN. If the task is within the legal limits of your role and in your job description, the RN can help you feel more comfortable with the task. The RN can answer your questions, demonstrate the task, show you how to use supplies and equipment, help you as needed, observe you performing the task, or check in on you often. The RN also can arrange for needed training.

With good communication, you and the RN should be able to work out the problem. If not, try talking to the RN's supervisor. When work problems continue, talk to someone whom you trust and can confide in. For example, your instructor or another professional can help you sort out work problems.

You must not refuse a delegated task simply because you do not like or want to do the task. You must have sound reasons for your refusal. Otherwise, you could place the patient at risk for harm. You also risk losing your job.

BOX 1-8 GUIDELINES FOR WORKING WITH THE NURSING AND HEALTH TEAMS

- Understand the roles, functions, and responsibilities in your job description.
- Make sure you are familiar with the personnel and procedure manuals.
- Report to work on time.
- Call the facility if you cannot report to work. Call as soon as possible, and give the reason for your absence.
- Practice good personal health and hygiene measures.
- Take pride in your appearance, and follow the facility's dress code.
- Act in an ethical and legal manner at all times.
- Treat patients, families, and co-workers with kindness and respect.
- Follow the RN's directions and instructions.
- Question unclear instructions and things you do not understand.

- Report patient complaints and your observations to the RN promptly.
- Help others willingly when asked.
- Offer to help others.
- Ask for additional tasks or activities during slow times.
- Do not waste supplies and equipment.
- Do not use the telephone, supplies, or equipment for your personal use.
- Follow the facility rules and regulations.
- Be accurate in measuring, reporting, and recording.
- Tell the RN when you are leaving and when you return to the nursing unit.
- Do not discuss your personal problems with patients or families.
- Ask for any training that you might need. ✳

WORK ETHICS

You work closely with RNs, LPNs/LVNs, assistive personnel, and other members of the health team. Acting in an ethically and legally responsible manner affects how you function, the quality of care you give, and your relationships with co-workers. The guidelines in Box 1-8 will help you work well with others.

Ethics deals with right and wrong conduct. It involves making choices and judgments about what or what not to do. An ethical person does the right thing. In the work place, certain behaviors (conduct), choices, and judgments are expected. Therefore **work ethics** deals with behavior in the workplace. Your conduct reflects your choices and judgments. Your appearance, what you say, how you behave, and how you treat and work with others are all part of work ethics. To get and keep a job, you must conduct yourself in the right way.

Preparing for Work

Having a job is a privilege. It is not a right or something due to you. You earned the job by getting the necessary education and training. You succeeded in a job interview. Now you must function well and work well with others to keep your job.

You must work when scheduled. This means getting to work on time and staying through the entire shift. Absences and tardiness (being late) are among the most common reasons for losing a job. Childcare and transportation issues often interfere with getting to work and getting to work on time. You need to plan in advance for childcare and transportation.

On the Job

You will have contact with patients, visitors, and co-workers. How you look, how you behave, and what you say affects everyone in the agency. Working when scheduled, being cheerful and friendly, performing delegated tasks, helping others, and being kind in what you do and say are part of good work ethics. OSF Saint Francis Medical Center's (Peoria, Ill.) *Employee Handbook* says it best:

You are what people see when they arrive here; yours are the eyes they look into when they're frightened and lonely. Yours are the voices people hear when they ride the elevators, when they try to sleep, and when they try to forget their problems. You are what they hear on their way to appointments which could affect their destinies, and what they hear after they leave those appointments. Yours are the comments people hear when you think they can't.

Yours is the intelligence and caring that people hope they'll find here. If you're noisy, so is the medical center. If you're rude, so is the medical center. And if you're wonderful, so is the medical center.

Attendance You must report to work when scheduled and on time. The entire unit is affected when just one person is late. You must call your supervisor if you will be late or cannot go to work. Attendance policies are explained in your employee handbook. You must follow these policies. Poor attendance can cause you to lose your job.

Being on time does not mean arriving at the facility when your shift begins. It means being ready to work when you shift starts. Remember, you need to store your coat, purse, backpack, or other personal items. You might need to use the restroom when you arrive at the facility. Plan to arrive on your nursing unit a few minutes early. This gives you time to greet others and settle yourself.

Attendance is more than getting to work when scheduled and on time. You must stay the entire shift. Preparing for childcare emergencies is important. Watching the clock as the shift ends gives a bad image. Working overtime is sometimes necessary. You need to prepare to stay longer if necessary.

focus on home care Home care assignments must be completed. You must never leave in the middle of an assignment. Nor should you leave before someone from the next shift arrives. Unfortunately, conflicts or problems may occur. Make every effort to finish the assignment. Explain the problem to your supervisor. The supervisor will try to make any needed changes. You must not walk out on the person. That would leave the person in an unsafe situation. Walking out is a most unethical behavior.

Your attitude You need to show a positive attitude about your job. Show that you are happy to be at the facility and that you enjoy your work. Listen to others, and be willing to learn. Stay busy, and use your time well.

The work you do is very important. RNs and patients rely on you to give good care. You need to believe that you and your work have value.

Always think before you speak. The following statements signal a negative attitude:

- "I can't. I'm too busy."
- "I didn't do it."
- "It's not my fault."
- "Don't blame me."
- "It's not my turn. I did it yesterday."
- "Nobody told me."
- "I can't come to work today. I have a headache."
- "That's not my job."
- "You didn't tell me that you needed it right away."
- "I work harder than anyone else."
- "No one appreciates what I do."

Gossip Gossip means spreading rumors or talking about the private matters of others. Gossiping is unprofessional. It can hurt others. The following guidelines will help you to avoid being a part of gossip:

- Remove yourself from a group or situation where gossip is occurring.
- Do not make or repeat any comment that can hurt a patient, family member, co-worker, or the facility.
- Do not make or repeat any comment that you do not know to be true. Remember, making or writing false statements about another person is defamation.
- Do not talk about patients, visitors, family members, co-workers, or the facility at home or in social settings.

Confidentiality Patient information is private and personal. **Confidentiality** means trusting others with personal and private information. Patient information is shared only among health team members involved in the person's care. Privacy and confidentiality are patient rights. Facility and co-worker information also is confidential.

Avoid talking about patients, the facility, or co-workers where others are present. Share information only with the RN supervising your work. Avoid talking about patients, the facility, or co-workers in hallways, elevators, dining areas, or outside the facility. Others not involved in the situation may overhear you. Patients and visitors are very alert to what is said. Other patients or visitors can overhear you and think you are talking about them or their loved ones. Misinformation and the wrong impressions are given about the patient's condition. You can easily upset the patient or family. Therefore you must be very careful about what you say, how you say it, when you say it, and where you say it.

Avoid eavesdropping. To eavesdrop means to listen in or overhear the conversations of others. When you eavesdrop, you invade another person's privacy.

Intercom systems require special considerations. Many facilities have intercom systems to allow communication between the bedside and the nurses' station. Patients use the intercom to signal when they need help. The intercom is answered by a staff member at the nurses' station. The nursing team also uses the intercom to communicate with other team members. Be careful what you say over the intercom. It is like a loud speaker. Others nearby can hear what you are saying.

Personal hygiene and appearance How you look affects the way people think about you and the agency. If staff are clean and neat, people think the facility is clean and neat. They think the facility is unclean if staff are messy and unkempt.

BOX 1-9 PRACTICES FOR A PROFESSIONAL APPEARANCE

- Uniforms fit well and are modest in length and style.

- Uniforms are clean, pressed, and mended. Wear a clean uniform daily.

- Wear your name badge or photo ID at all times when on duty.

- Underclothes are clean and fit properly. They are changed daily and are an appropriate color. Colored undergarments can be seen through white and light colored uniforms.

- Jewelry is not worn. Most agencies let employees wear wedding rings; some allow engagement rings. Large rings and bracelets can scratch patients. Confused or combative persons can easily pull off necklaces, bracelets, and earrings. Young children also like to pull on jewelry.

- Stockings or socks are clean, well-fitting, and changed daily.

- Shoes are comfortable, give needed support, and fit properly. Clean and polish shoes often. Wash laces, and replace them as necessary.

- Fingernails are clean, short, and neatly shaped.

- Nail polish is not worn. Chipped nail polish provides a place for microorganisms to grow and multiply.

- Hairstyles are simple and attractive. Hair is off your collar and away from your face. Use simple pins, combs, barrettes, and bands to keep long hair up and in place.

- Makeup is modest in amount and moderate in color. Avoid a painted and severe appearance.

- Perfume, cologne, and after-shave lotions are not worn. They may offend and nauseate patients. ✳

Attire that is accepted in home and social settings is often unacceptable in the work setting. You cannot wear jeans, halter tops, tank tops, or short skirts. Clothing must not be sexual in nature. That is, females cannot show cleavage, the tops of breasts, or the upper thigh. Males must avoid tight pants and exposing their chests. Only the top shirt button can be open.

Follow these guidelines for good personal hygiene and appearance in the work setting:

- Practice personal hygiene.

- Follow the guideline for professional appearance listed in Box 1-9.

- Follow the facility's dress code.

- Tend to grooming needs in private. Use the restroom to brush hair, freshen make-up, apply lipstick, floss, or brush your teeth.

- Do not chew gum, smoke, or chew tobacco while on duty.

- Cover tattoos. They may offend patients, visitors, and co-workers.

Speech and language Your speech and language must be professional. Accepted speech and language in home and social settings may be unacceptable at work. The words you use when talking to family and friends may offend patients, visitors, and co-workers. Remember the following:

- Do not swear or use foul, vulgar, or abusive language.

- Do not use slang.

- Control the volume and tone of your voice. Speak softly and gently.

- Speak clearly. Persons with hearing problems may have difficulty hearing you.

- Do not shout or yell.

- Do not fight or argue with patients, families, or co-workers.

Courtesies A **courtesy** is a polite, considerate, or helpful comment or act. Courtesies are easy. They require little time or energy. And they mean so much to people. Even the smallest act of kindness can brighten someone's day:

- Address others by Miss, Mrs., Ms., Mr., or Doctor. Call a person by first name only if he or she asks you to do so.

- Say "please." Begin or end each request with "please."

- Say "thank you" whenever someone does something for you.

- Apologize to others. Say "I'm sorry" whenever you make a mistake or hurt someone. Even little things—like bumping into someone in the hallway—require an apology.

- Be thoughtful of others. Compliment others as appropriate. Wish others a happy birthday, a happy day or weekend off, or a happy holiday.

- Wish patients and families well when they leave the agency. "Stay well" or "stay healthy" are good phrases to use.

- Hold doors open for others. If you are at the door first, open the door and let others pass through. In business, males and females hold doors open for each other.

- Hold elevator doors open for others coming down the hallway.

- Help others willingly when asked.

- Praise others. If you see a co-worker do or say something that impresses you, tell that person. Also tell your co-workers.

- Do not take credit for another person's deed. Give the person credit for the action.

Personal matters You are employed to do a job. Personal matters cannot interfere with the job. Otherwise patient care is neglected. You could lose your job for tending to personal matters while at work. Practice the following to keep personal matters separate from the work place:

- Make personal phone calls only during breaks and lunch. Use public pay phones.

- Do not let family and friends visit you on the unit. If they must see you, arrange for them to meet you for lunch.

- Arrange personal appointments (doctor, dentist, lawyer, beauty, and others) for times when you are not scheduled to work.

- Do not use facility computers, printers, fax machines, or photocopiers for your personal use.

- Do not take facility supplies (pens, paper, and others) for your personal use.

- Do not discuss personal problems at work.

- Control your emotions. If you need to cry or express anger, do so in a private place. Get yourself together quickly, and return to your work.

- Avoid borrowing money from or lending money to co-workers. This includes lunch money and bus or train fares. Borrowing and lending can lead to problems with co-workers.

- Do not engage in fund-raising activities at work. Do not sell your child's candy or raffle tickets to co-workers.

- Do not carry personal pagers or cellular phones while at work.

Lunches and breaks Everyone has a lunch time and two breaks during an 8-hour shift. The lunch break is usually 30 minutes long. Breaks are usually for 15 minutes. Lunches and breaks are scheduled so that some staff are always on the unit. Staff remaining on the unit cover for the staff on break.

Staff members have responsibilities to each other. Leave for and return from your break on time. That way other staff can have their breaks. Do not take longer than you are allowed. Also remember to tell the RN when you leave and return to the unit.

Job safety Safety involves protecting patients, visitors, co-workers, and yourself from harm. Every employee is responsible for job safety. Negligent behavior affects the safety of others. Safety practices are presented throughout this book. The following guidelines are important no matter what you are doing:

- Understand the roles, functions, and responsibilities in your job description.

- Be familiar with the contents and policies in personnel and procedure manuals.

- Know the difference between right and wrong.

- Know what you can and cannot do.

- Develop the desired qualities and characteristics of assistive personnel.

- Follow the RN's directions and instructions.

BOX 1-10 PLANNING AND ORGANIZING YOUR WORK

- Discuss priorities with the RN.
- Know the routine of your shift and nursing unit.
- List care or procedures that are on a schedule. Some persons are turned or offered the bedpan every 2 hours.
- Estimate how much time is needed for each person, procedure, and task.
- Identify which tasks and procedures can be done while patients are eating, visiting, or involved in activities or therapies.
- Plan care around meal times, visiting hours, and therapies. If working in a long-term care center, you must also consider daily recreation and social activities.

- Identify situations in which you will need help from a co-worker. Ask a co-worker to help you, and give the approximate time when you will need help.
- Schedule any equipment or rooms if necessary. Some facilities have only one shower or bathtub to a nursing unit. You will need to schedule the room for patient use.
- Review the procedures to be performed, and gather needed supplies beforehand.
- Do not waste time. Stay focused on your work.
- Do not leave a messy work area. Make sure patient rooms are neat and orderly. Also clean utility areas.
- Be a self-starter. That is, have initiative. Ask others if they need help, follow unit routines, stock supply areas, and clean utility rooms. Stay busy. ✳

- Question unclear instructions and things you do not understand.
- Help others willingly when asked.
- Follow facility rules and regulations.
- Ask for any training that you might need.
- Report measurements, observations, the care given, patient complaints, and any errors accurately.
- Accept responsibility for your actions. Admit when you are wrong or make mistakes. Do not blame others. Do not make excuses for your actions.

Planning and organizing your work Working well with others includes working in an organized and efficient way. You will give nursing care to patients. You also will perform routine tasks on the nursing unit. Some assignments must be completed by a certain time. Other tasks or functions are to be done by the end of the shift. You must plan and organize your work to give safe, thorough care and to make good use of your time. The guidelines in Box 1-10 will help you plan and organize your work.

HARASSMENT

Harassment means troubling, tormenting, offending, or worrying a person by one's behavior or comments. Harassment can be sexual. Or it can involve one's age, race, ethnic background, religion, or disability. What you say and do must be respectful of others. You must not offend others by your gestures, remarks, or use of touch. Nor can you offend others with jokes or pictures. Harassment is not legal in the workplace.

Sexual Harassment

Sexual harassment involves unwanted sexual behaviors by another. The behavior may be a sexual advance or request for a sexual favor. It can be in the form of a comment or touch. The behavior interferes with the person's work and comfort. In extreme cases, the person's job may be threatened if sexual favors are not granted.

Victims of sexual harassment may be men or women. Men harass women or men. Women harass men or women. If you feel that you are being harassed, you must report the situation to your supervisor and the human resource officer.

BOX 1-11   COMMON REASONS FOR LOSING A JOB

- Poor attendance—not showing up for work or excessive tardiness (being late)
- Abandonment—leaving the job during your shift
- Falsifying a record—application or patient record
- Violent behavior in the workplace
- Possessing weapons in the work setting—guns, knives, explosives, or other dangerous items
- Possessing, using, or distributing alcohol in the work setting
- Possessing, using, or distributing illegal/controlled drugs in the work setting (this excludes taking drugs ordered by a doctor)
- Taking a patient's drug for your own use or distribution to others
- Harassment—see p. 17
- Using offensive speech and language

- Stealing the facility's or a patient's property
- Destroying the facility's or a patient's property
- Showing disrespect to patients, visitors, co-workers, or supervisors
- Abusing or neglecting a patient
- Invading a person's privacy
- Failing to maintain patient, facility, or co-worker confidentiality (includes access to computer information)
- Using the employer's supplies and equipment for your own use
- Abusing lunch and break periods
- Sleeping on the job
- Violating facility dress code
- Violating any facility policy
- Tending to personal matters while on duty ✳

You must be careful about what you say or do. Even innocent remarks and behaviors can be viewed as harassment. Employee orientation programs include information about harassment. If you are not sure about your own or another person's remarks or behaviors, discuss the situation with the RN. You cannot be too careful.

LOSING A JOB

Remember, a job is a privilege. You must perform your job well and protect patients from harm. Not being awarded a pay raise or losing your job results from poor performance. Failure to follow a facility policy is often grounds for termination. So is failure to get along with others. Box 1-11 lists the many reasons why you can lose your job. Protect your job by performing to the best of your ability. Always practice good work ethics.

SUMMARY

More and more hospitals are using assistive personnel to assist nurses with patient care. The roles, functions, and responsibilities of assistive personnel vary from state to state and among facilities. The state's nurse practice act provides the framework for the tasks that RNs can delegate to assistive personnel. Your job description should include only those tasks allowed by your state. Also, you should have the necessary training to perform the task.

RNs use the five rights of delegation when making delegation decisions. The five rights are the right task, the right circumstances, the right person, the right directions and communication, and the right supervision. Delegation decisions should always be in the best interests of the person. The person's health and safety must be protected.

You should also use the five rights when deciding to accept or to refuse a delegated task. If you accept a delegated task, you are responsible for completing the task safely. If you need to refuse a delegated task, you must communicate your concerns to the RN. Patient care cannot be neglected.

Your work is important to patients, RNs, and the health team. How you behave affects everyone. You must conduct yourself in an ethical manner. Getting to work when scheduled and on time is important. Your attitude, appearance, and speech and language tell a lot about you. So do the courtesies you show others. Remember not to gossip. Always keep patient and employee information confidential. Tend to personal matters on your own time.

REVIEW QUESTIONS

Circle T *if the answer is true and* F *if the answer is false.*

1 T F Childcare and transportation issues require planning before going to work.

2 T F Being on time for work means arriving at your facility when your shift begins.

3 T F Failure to maintain confidentiality is grounds for losing your job.

4 T F You must be careful what you say over the intercom system.

5 T F You can use the facility's computer for your personal use.

6 T F You should carry a personal pager so family members can reach you.

7 T F Harassment is legal in the workplace.

Circle the best *answer.*

8 The increased use of assistive personnel is a result of
a Primary nursing
b Team nursing
c Rising health care costs
d Patients being quite ill

9 Which health care trend moves patient services from departments to the bedside?
a Managed care
b Health care systems
c Staffing mix
d Patient-focused care

10 Nursing practice is regulated by
a OBRA
b Medicare and Medicaid
c Nurse practice acts
d All of the above

REVIEW QUESTIONS—CONT'D

11 OBRA sets training and competency evaluation standards for assistive personnel working in
  a Home care
  b Hospitals
  c Long-term care
  d All of the above

12 What state law affects what assistive personnel can do?
  a The state's nurse practice act
  b OBRA
  c Medicare
  d Medicaid

13 You perform a nursing task not allowed by your state. Which is *true*?
  a If an RN delegated the task, there is no legal problem.
  b You could be found guilty of practicing nursing without a license.
  c Performing the task is allowed if it is in your job description.
  d If you complete the task safely, there is no legal problem.

14 An RN asks you to give medications. Which is *true*?
  a Assistive personnel never give medications.
  b The RN must supervise your work.
  c You must be trained to give medications.
  d You must know how the medications affect the patient.

15 These statements are about delegation. Which is *false*?
  a RNs can delegate their responsibilities to you.
  b A delegated task must be safe for the patient.
  c The delegated task must be in your job description.
  d The delegating nurse is responsible for the safe completion of the task.

16 A task is in your job description. Which is *false*?
  a The RN must always delegate the task to you.
  b The RN delegates the task to you if the patient's circumstances are right.
  c The RN must make sure you have the necessary education and training.
  d You must have clear directions before you perform the task.

17 An RN delegates a task to you. You must
  a Complete the task
  b Decide if you can accept the task or if you must say "no"
  c Delegate the task to another assistive person if you are too busy to complete the task
  d Ignore the request if you do not know how to perform the task

18 You are responsible for
  a Completing tasks safely
  b Delegation
  c The "five rights of delegation"
  d Delegating tasks to assistive personnel

19 You can refuse to perform a task for the following reasons *except*
  a The task is beyond the legal limits of your role
  b The task is not in your job description
  c You do not like the task
  d An RN is not available to supervise you

20 When you refuse to perform a task, your first action is to
  a Delegate the task to another assistive person
  b Communicate your concerns to the RN
  c Ignore the request
  d Talk to the RN's supervisor

21 When working with others, you must do the following *except*
  a Help others only when asked
  b Report to work on time
  c Ask for other tasks or activities during slow times
  d Report observations and patient complaints to the RN

22 Which statement reflects a positive work attitude?
  a "It's not my fault."
  b "Please show me how this works."
  c "That's not my job."
  d "I did it yesterday. It's her turn."

23 A co-worker tells you that a doctor and nurse are dating. This is
  a Gossip
  b Eavesdropping
  c Confidential information
  d Sexual harassment

REVIEW QUESTIONS—CONT'D

24 Which is professional speech and language?
   a Speaking clearly
   b Using vulgar and abusive words
   c Shouting
   d Arguing

25 Which is *not* a courteous act?
   a Saying "please" and "thank you"
   b Expecting others to open doors for you
   c Saying "I'm sorry"
   d Complimenting others

26 You are on your lunch break. Which is *false*?
   a You can make personal phone calls.
   b Family members can meet you for lunch.
   c You can take a few extra minutes if necessary.
   d The RN needs to know that you are off the unit.

27 You are organizing your work. You should do the following *except*
   a Discuss priorities with the RN
   b Ask others if they need help
   c Stay busy
   d Plan care so that you can watch the patient's TV

Answers to these questions are on p. 179

2 *Surgical Asepsis*

OBJECTIVES

- Define the key terms in this chapter
- Explain the principles and practices of surgical asepsis
- Explain how to open sterile packages and pour sterile solutions
- Explain how to set up a sterile field
- Describe how to handle sterile forceps with and without sterile gloves
- Describe what you can touch when donning and wearing sterile gloves
- Perform the procedures described in this chapter

KEY TERMS

contamination The process by which an object or area becomes unclean

nonpathogen A microorganism that does not usually cause an infection

normal flora Microorganisms that usually live and grow in a certain location

pathogen A microorganism that causes an infection and is harmful

sterile The absence of all microorganisms

sterile field A work area free of all pathogens and nonpathogens

sterile technique Surgical asepsis

surgical asepsis The practices that keep equipment and supplies free of all microorganisms; sterile technique

Surgical asepsis (sterile technique) is the practice that keeps equipment and supplies free of all microorganisms (microbes). **Sterile** means the absence of *all* microbes. Some microbes cause infections and are considered harmful. They are called **pathogens. Nonpathogens** are microbes that do not usually cause an infection.

Normal flora are microbes that usually live and grow in a certain area. Certain microbes are found in the respiratory tract, in the intestines, and on the skin. They are nonpathogens when in or on a natural reservoir. When a nonpathogen is transmitted from its natural site to another site or host, it becomes a pathogen. *Escherichia coli* is normally found in the large intestine. If the *E. coli* enters the urinary system, it can cause an infection.

Surgical asepsis is required for any procedure that involves penetrating the skin or sterile tissues. The operating room and labor and delivery areas require surgical asepsis. Many diagnostic and nursing procedures also require surgical asepsis. If any break occurs in sterile technique, pathogens and nonpathogens can enter the person's body and cause an infection.

PRINCIPLES OF SURGICAL ASEPSIS

Operating room and labor and delivery personnel must follow certain procedures. A mask and surgical cap are worn for hand washing. This hand washing is called a surgical "scrub" and takes at least 5 minutes. Then a sterile gown and sterile gloves are put on. When you perform or assist with a sterile procedure at the bedside, regular hand washing and sterile gloves are needed. Personal protective equipment (gown, mask, and goggles or eye shield) are worn as needed to prevent contact with blood, body fluids, secretions, and excretions.

When performing a sterile procedure, all items in contact with the person must be kept sterile. If any item becomes contaminated, the person is at risk for infection. (**Contamination** is the process by which an object or area becomes unclean. A sterile item or area is contaminated whenever microbes are on the item or area). Therefore a sterile field must be maintained. A **sterile field** is a work area free of pathogenic and nonpathogenic microorganisms. Box 2-1 on p. 24 lists the principles and practices of surgical asepsis that are followed in maintaining a sterile field and in performing a sterile procedure.

focus on home care You may need to clean an area or surface in the home before you practice surgical asepsis. Practice Standard Precautions, and clean the work surface with soap and water. Remember to clean from the cleanest area to the dirtiest. Also clean away from your body and uniform. Dry the surface after cleaning.

BOX 2-1 PRINCIPLES AND PRACTICES FOR SURGICAL ASEPSIS

- A sterile item can be touched only by another sterile item:
  * If a sterile item touches a clean item, the sterile item is contaminated.
  * If a clean item touches a sterile item, the sterile item is contaminated.
  * A sterile package that is open, torn, punctured, wet, or moist is contaminated.
  * A sterile package is contaminated after the expiration date on the package.
  * Place only sterile items on a sterile field.
  * Use sterile gloves or sterile forceps to handle other sterile items (Fig. 2-1).
  * Consider any item to be contaminated if you are unsure of its sterility.
  * Contaminated items are not used. They are discarded or resterilized.

- Sterile items or a sterile field must always be within your vision and above your waist:
  * If you cannot see an item, the item is contaminated.
  * If the item is below your waist, the item is contaminated.
  * Keep sterile gloved hands above your waist and within your sight.
  * Do not leave a sterile field unattended.
  * Do not turn your back on a sterile field.

- Airborne microorganisms can contaminate sterile items or a sterile field:
  * Prevent drafts by closing the door and avoiding excessive movements. Other personnel in the room should also avoid excessive moving.
  * Avoid coughing, sneezing, talking, or laughing over a sterile field. Turn your head away from the sterile field if you must talk.

  * Wear mask if you need to talk during the procedure.
  * Do not perform sterile procedures if you have a respiratory infection.
  * Do not reach over a sterile field.

- Fluid flows downward, in the direction of gravity:
  * Hold wet items down (see Fig. 2-1). If held up, fluid can flow down into a contaminated area. The contaminated fluid flows back into the sterile field when the item is held down.
  * Hold your hands higher than your elbows during a surgical scrub. Water from your elbows will not flow onto your clean hands and fingers.

- The sterile field must be kept dry, unless the area below it is sterile:
  * The sterile field is contaminated if it becomes wet and the area below it is not sterile.
  * Avoid spilling and splashing when pouring sterile fluids into sterile containers.

- The edges of a sterile field are contaminated:
  * A 1-inch (2.5-cm) margin around the sterile field is contaminated (Fig. 2-2).
  * Place all sterile items inside the 1-inch (2.5-cm) margin of the sterile field.
  * Items outside the 1-inch (2.5-cm) margin are contaminated.

- Honesty is essential to sterile technique:
  * You know when you contaminate an item or sterile field. Be honest with yourself even if no other staff members are present.
  * Remove the contaminated item and correct the situation. You may need to start over with sterile supplies.
  * Report the contamination to the RN. ※

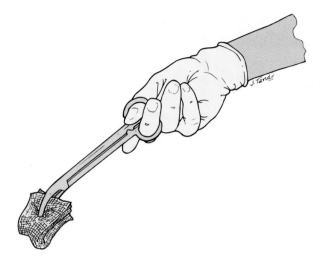

Fig. 2-1 *Sterile forceps are used to handle sterile items.*

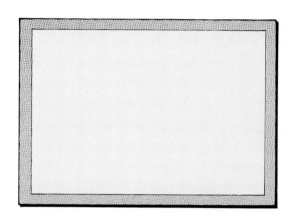

Fig. 2-2 *A 1-inch (2.5-cm) margin around the sterile field is considered contaminated.*

STERILE EQUIPMENT AND SUPPLIES

Sterile equipment and supplies are wrapped in cloth, paper, or plastic. Sterile liquids are sealed in containers. Labeling indicates that the item is sterile. Some items have a chemical tape that changes color when sterilized. In addition, each item is marked with an expiration date. If the date is past, do not use the item. If the seal is broken on a container, do not use the solution. When handling sterile equipment and supplies, you must follow the principles and practices listed in Box 2-1. Also make sure that you wash your hands before opening sterile items and establishing a sterile field.

Opening Sterile Packages

Sterile packages are wrapped and have four flaps or corners. Other packages are peel-back. Different techniques are used to open wrapped and peel-back packages. Opening wrapped packages on a surface and while holding them also require different techniques.

No matter what type of packaging, the inside of a sterile package is sterile and is a sterile field. Before opening a sterile package, make sure the package is intact. The package must be dry and free of tears, punctures, holes, and watermarks. *Do not open sterile packages while wearing sterile gloves. The outside of the package is unsterile. You will contaminate your gloves.*

OPENING A STERILE PACKAGE

PRE-PROCEDURE

1 Wash your hands.

2 Make sure you have all needed supplies and equipment.

3 Inspect the package to ensure sterility:

a Check labeling and the chemical tape for sterility.

b Check the expiration date.

c Make sure the package is dry.

d Check the package for tears, holes, punctures, and watermarks.

4 Prepare the person for the procedure:

a Explain the procedure to the person.

b Check ID bracelet. Identify the person with the assignment sheet.

c Provide for the person's privacy. Close the door, and pull the privacy curtain.

d Assist the person to meet elimination needs.

e Wash your hands.

f Drape the person for the procedure and for privacy.

5 Arrange a work surface.

a Make sure you will have enough room.

b Arrange the work surface at waist level and within your vision. Make sure you will not have to reach over or turn your back on the work surface.

c Clean and dry the work surface.

PROCEDURE

6 Opening a wrapped sterile package on a surface:

a Place the sterile package in the center of your work surface.

b Position the package so the top flap points toward you.

c Reach around the package, and grasp the outside of the top flap with your thumb and index finger (Fig. 2-3, *A*).

d Pull the flap open, and lay it flat.

e Grasp the outside of the first side flap with your thumb and index finger. Use your right hand if the flap is on your right and your left hand if it is on your left. Pull the flap open, and lay it flat (Fig. 2-3, *B*).

f Repeat step 6-e for the other side flap (Fig. 2-3, *C*).

g Grasp the outside of the fourth flap. Stand back and away from the package, and pull the flap back (Fig. 2-3, *D*). Let the flap lay flat. Make sure the flap does not touch your uniform or any contaminated surface.

h Remember that the 1-inch (2.5-cm) margin on the inside of the wrapper is contaminated (see Fig. 2-2). The rest of the inside wrapper is sterile. Do not let any contaminated item touch this area.

7 Opening a wrapped sterile package while holding it (Fig. 2-4):

a Hold the package in your left hand if you are right-handed and in your right hand if you are left-handed.

b Hold the package so that the top flap points toward you.

c Reach behind the top flap and open it away from you.

d Open each side flap away from the package.

e Open the fourth flap toward you.

f Make sure your hands do not touch the inside wrapper or the package contents.

g Hold the package so the RN can grasp the contents. The RN wears sterile gloves.

h Do the following to transfer the package contents to a sterile field:

1) Hold the package wrapper back and away from the sterile field (Fig. 2-5, *A*, p. 28).

2) Drop the contents onto the sterile field (Fig. 2-5, *B*, p. 28).

8 Opening a peel-back package:

a Read the package instructions.

b Two flaps: grasp the two flaps, and gently peel the flaps back (Fig. 2-6, p. 28).

c One flap: hold the package, and pull back the flap (Fig. 2-7, p. 28).

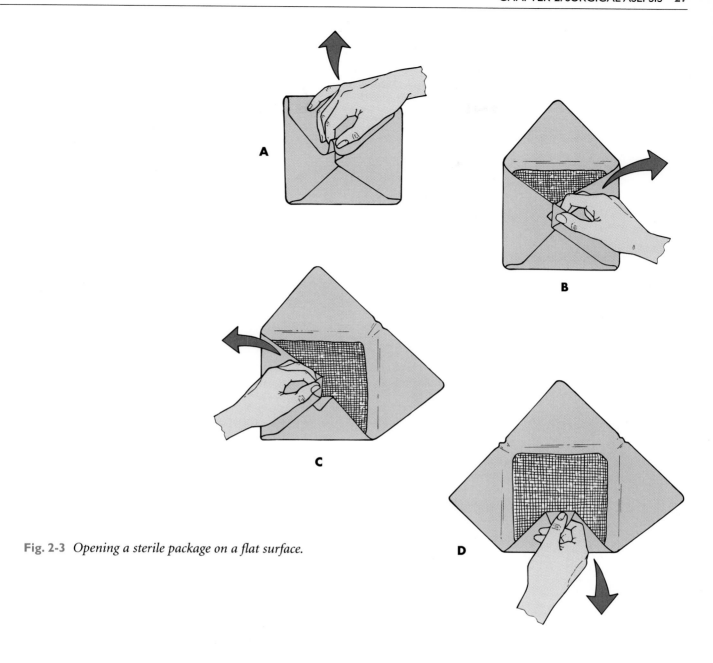

Fig. 2-3 *Opening a sterile package on a flat surface.*

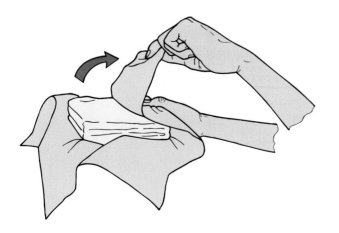

Fig. 2-4 *Opening a sterile package while holding it. Note that package is held away from the person so that the wrapper is not contaminated.*

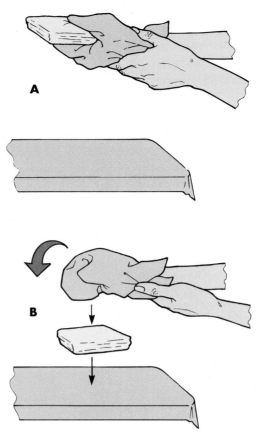

Fig. 2-5 *Transferring package contents to a sterile field.* **A,** *Hold the wrapper back after opening the package.* **B,** *Drop the contents onto the sterile field.*

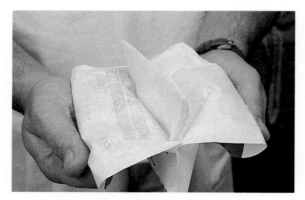

Fig. 2-6 *The flaps of a peel-back package are carefully peeled back.*

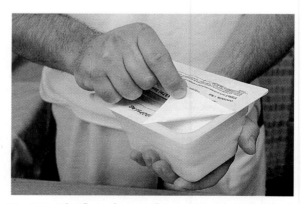

Fig. 2-7 *The flap of a one-flap package is pulled back.*

Opening and Pouring Sterile Solutions

Sterile solutions are usually obtained from the supply department. The solution container is sealed. The outside of the container and cap is unsterile. The inside of the cap and bottle is sterile.

Inspect the container when collecting your supplies. Make sure the container is not cracked or broken. Also make sure that the seal is intact. Return the bottle to the supply department if the bottle is cracked or broken or if the seal is broken.

Some sterile packages contain sterile solutions. These containers are opened while wearing sterile gloves.

Sterile solutions are poured into sterile containers. Do not pour a sterile solution into a clean container. This contaminates the sterile solution.

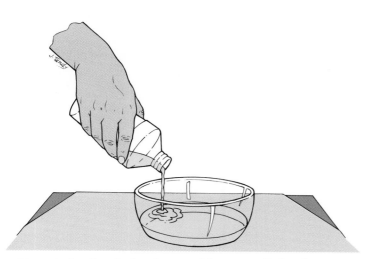

Fig. 2-8 *Sterile solution is poured into a sterile bowl. Care is taken to avoid spills or splashing.*

OPENING AND POURING A STERILE SOLUTION

PRE-PROCEDURE

1 Obtain the correct solution.
2 Inspect the container for cracks and breaks.
3 Make sure the seal is unbroken.

PROCEDURE

4 Hold the container so the label is in your palm. This protects the label from becoming wet from dripping solution.
5 Twist off the cap to break the seal.
6 Place the cap, inside up, on a clean surface.
7 Hold the container 4 to 6 inches over the sterile bowl (Fig. 2-8). Make sure the container does not touch the sterile bowl.
8 Pour the solution into the sterile bowl. Pour slowly to avoid splashing.

POST-PROCEDURE

9 Recap the container. Discard the container if it is empty or remaining solution will not be used:
10 Do the following if remaining solution will be used:
   a Make sure the remaining solution was not contaminated.
   b Label the container with the person's name, the date, and the time.
   c Store the container following facility policy.

SETTING UP A STERILE FIELD

The sterile field provides a sterile work area. Once the sterile field is set up, you can add other sterile items to the field. The inside wrapper of a sterile package or a sterile drape can be used. Drapes often provide larger sterile fields than the inside of the sterile package.

A sterile drape is contained within sterile packaging. You open the package as described earlier. Remember, the inside 1-inch (2.5-cm) margin of the drape is contaminated.

SETTING UP A STERILE FIELD

PROCEDURE

1 Follow Pre-procedure steps listed in *Opening a Sterile Package*.

2 Open the sterile package (see *Opening a Sterile Package*).

3 Pick up the folded top edge of the drape with your thumb and index finger.

4 Remove the drape from the package. Lift it away from you and allow it to unfold (Fig. 2-9, *A*). Discard the packaging.

5 Make sure the drape does not touch your uniform, the outer packaging, or any other surface.

6 Pick up the other corner of the drape. Make sure you hold the drape away from you and other contaminated surfaces.

7 Lay the drape on your work surface (Fig. 2-9, *B*). Start with the bottom half (the side away from you).

8 Add other sterile items to the sterile field as necessary:

   a Open each sterile package.

   b Hold the package wrapper back and away from the sterile field.

   c Drop the contents onto the sterile field or use a transfer forceps.

Using a Transfer Forceps

Forceps are instruments used to pick up, hold, and transfer items (see Fig. 2-1). Sterile forceps are used to transfer sterile items to or within a sterile field. They are used also for handling sterile items during a procedure. They are resterilized after use. You need to remember the following when using sterile forceps:

- Hold sterile forceps above your waist.

- Hold wet forceps so the tips are lower than your wrist.

- Keep sterile forceps within your sight.

- Make sure the forceps do not touch the outside of any packaging.

- Make sure the forceps do not touch the 1-inch (2.5-cm) margin around the drape.

- Lay the forceps down carefully within the sterile field.

  * Not wearing sterile gloves: lay the tips within the sterile field and the handles outside the sterile field.

  * Wearing sterile gloves: lay the entire forceps within the sterile field.

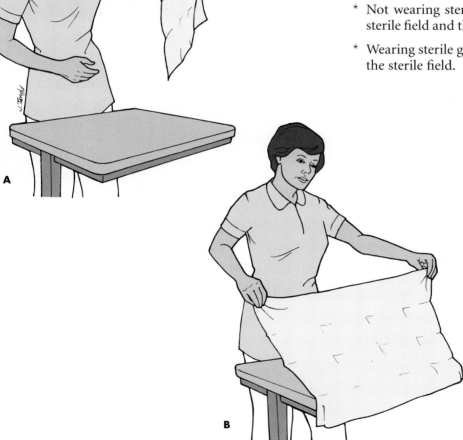

Fig. 2-9 *Opening a sterile drape.* **A,** *The drape is held by a corner and allowed to open freely.* **B,** *The drape is placed over a work surface. Note that it is held at two corners.*

DONNING AND REMOVING STERILE GLOVES

Sterile gloves are put on after the sterile field is set up. After putting on sterile gloves, you can handle sterile items within the sterile field. You cannot touch anything outside the sterile field.

In operating rooms and delivery areas, the closed method of sterile gloving is followed. A sterile gown is donned and then the sterile gloves. The procedure is called *closed gloving* because you put on the gloves while your hands are inside the gown cuffs. You will learn sterile gowning and the closed gloving method if you work in those areas. The open method of gloving is used for sterile procedures at the bedside. It is called the *open method* because your hands are not covered by gown cuffs.

Sterile gloves are disposable and are supplied in peel-back packaging. They come in a variety of sizes so that they fit snugly. The insides are powdered for ease in donning the gloves. In addition, the packaging identifies the right and left glove.

Remember to keep sterile-gloved hands above your waist and within your vision. Also, you can touch only items within the sterile field. If at any time your gloves become contaminated, you must remove the gloves and put on a new pair. Also, replace gloves that are torn, cut, or punctured.

DONNING AND REMOVING STERILE GLOVES

PROCEDURE

1 Follow Pre-procedure steps listed in *Opening a Sterile Package.*

2 Open the package of sterile gloves using the peel-back method.

3 Remove the inner package. Place it on a clean work surface. Make sure the work surface is at waist height.

4 Read any manufacturer's instructions or information on the inner packaging. The packaging may be labeled with left, right, up, and down.

5 Arrange the inner package for left, right, up, and down. Make sure that the left glove will be on your left and the right glove on your right. The cuffs should be near you with the fingers pointing away.

6 Use the thumb and index finger of each hand to grasp the folded edges of the inner packaging.

7 Fold back the inner packaging to expose the gloves (Fig. 2-10, *A*). Do not touch or otherwise contaminate the inside of the package or the gloves. The inside of the inner package is a sterile field.

8 Note that each glove has a cuff about 2 to 3 inches wide. The cuffs and insides of the gloves are not considered sterile.

9 Put on the right glove if you are right-handed. Put on the left glove if you are left-handed:

   a Pick up the glove with your other hand. Use your thumb and index and middle fingers (Fig. 2-10, *B*).

   b Touch only the cuff and the inside of the glove.

   c Turn the hand to be gloved palm side up.

   d Lift the cuff up and slide your fingers and hand into the glove (Fig. 2-10, *C*).

   e Pull the glove up over your hand. If some fingers get stuck, leave them that way until the other glove is on. *Do not use your ungloved hand to straighten the glove. Do not let the outside of the glove touch any nonsterile surface.*

   f Leave the cuff turned down.

10 Put on the other glove with your gloved hand:

   a Reach under the cuff of the second glove with the four fingers of your gloved hand (Fig. 2-10, *D*). Keep your gloved thumb close to your gloved palm.

   b Pull on the second glove (Fig. 2-10, *E*). Your gloved hand cannot touch the cuff or any other surface. Hold the thumb of your first gloved hand away from your gloved palm.

11 Adjust each glove with the other hand. The gloves should be smooth and comfortable (Fig. 2-10, *F*).

12 Slide your fingers under the cuffs to pull them up (Fig. 2-10, *G*).

13 Touch only sterile items.

14 Remove the gloves as in Figure 2-11 on p. 34.

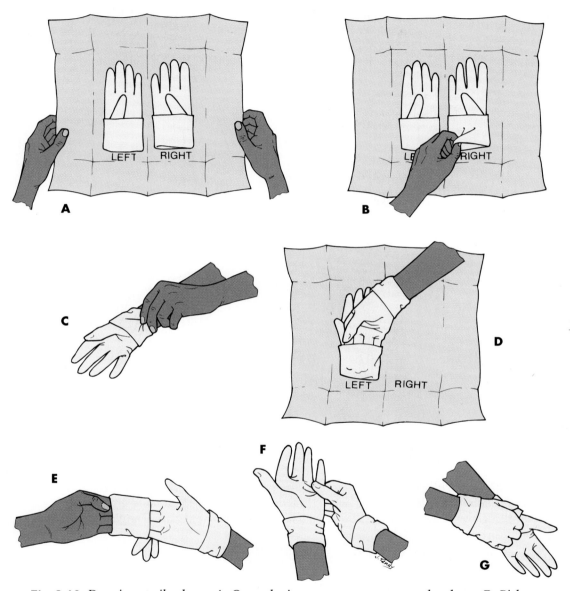

Fig. 2-10 *Donning sterile gloves.* **A,** *Open the inner wrapper to expose the gloves.* **B,** *Pick up the glove at the cuff with your thumb and index finger.* **C,** *Slide your fingers and hand into the glove.* **D,** *Reach under the cuff of the other glove with your fingers.* **E,** *Pull on the glove.* **F,** *Adjust each glove for comfort.* **G,** *Slide your fingers under the cuffs to pull them up.*

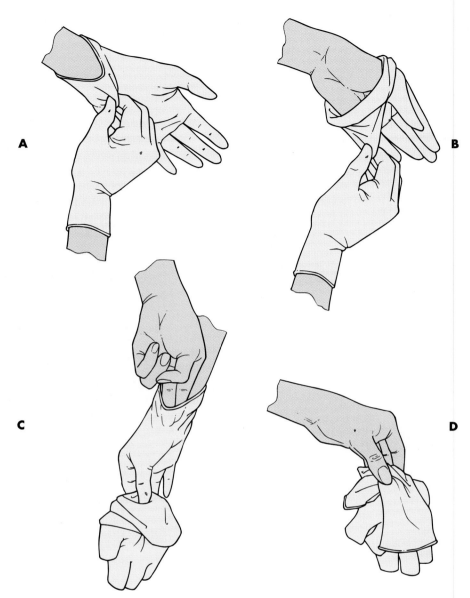

Fig. 2-11 *Removing gloves. **A,** The glove is grasped below the cuff. **B,** The glove is pulled down over the hand. The glove is inside out. **C,** The fingers of the ungloved hand are inserted inside the other glove. **D,** The glove is pulled down and over the hand and glove. The glove is inside out.*

SUMMARY

Surgical asepsis involves the absence of all microbes—pathogens and nonpathogens. You use the sterile procedures in this chapter when catheterizing persons and changing sterile dressings. Preventing contamination is important. Microbes must not enter sterile body areas. Otherwise, the person is at risk for infection. If you contaminate a sterile field or a sterile object, you must remove the contaminated item. Start over if necessary. Remember, honesty is an essential part of sterile technique.

REVIEW QUESTIONS

Circle T *if the answer is true and* F *if the answer is false.*

1 T F An item is sterile if nonpathogens are present.

2 T F The 1-inch (2.5-cm) edge around a sterile field is contaminated.

3 T F A sterile package has a watermark. The package is contaminated.

4 T F Sterile gloves are worn to set up a sterile field.

5 T F The inside and cuffs of sterile gloves are considered contaminated.

6 T F A sterile item can touch only another sterile item.

7 T F Wet items are held up.

8 T F If you cannot see an item, it is contaminated.

9 T F Sterile items must be kept above your waist.

10 T F You opened a container of sterile solution. The cap is held in your hand.

11 T F Forceps are held above your waist and kept within your sight.

12 T F Forceps are held so the tips are lower than your wrist.

13 T F Forceps must always be held with sterile gloved hands.

14 T F Forceps cannot touch the outside of any packaging.

Answers to these questions are on p. 179

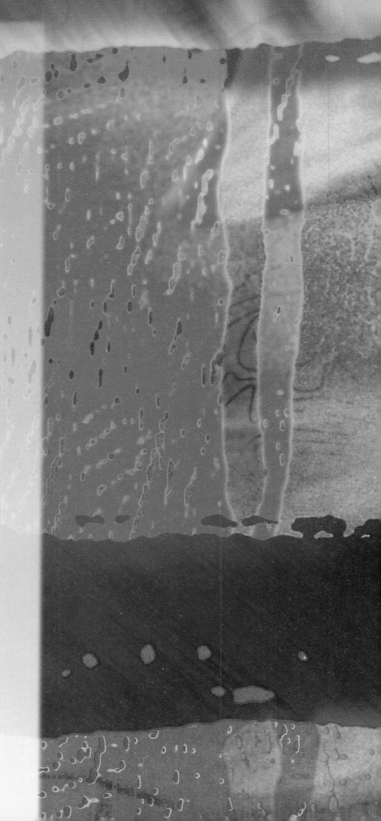

3

Assisting With Wound Care

OBJECTIVES

- Define the key terms in this chapter
- Describe the different types of wounds
- Describe the process, types, and complications of wound healing
- Describe the observations to make about a wound
- Describe the different types of wound drainage
- Explain how to measure wound drainage
- Explain how to secure dressings
- Explain the rules for applying dressings
- Explain the rules for cleaning wounds and drain sites
- Explain the purpose of binders and how to apply them
- Describe how to meet the basic needs of persons with wounds
- Perform the procedures described in this chapter

KEY TERMS

abrasion A partial-thickness wound caused by the scraping away or rubbing of the skin

chronic wound A wound that does not heal easily

clean wound A wound that is not infected

clean-contaminated wound A wound occurring from the surgical entry of the urinary, reproductive, respiratory, or gastrointestinal system

closed wound A wound in which tissues are injured but the skin is not broken

contaminated wound A wound with a high risk of infection

contusion A closed wound caused by a blow to the body

dehiscence The separation of wound layers

dirty wound An infected wound

evisceration The separation of the wound along with the protrusion of abdominal organs

full-thickness wound The dermis, epidermis, and subcutaneous tissue are penetrated; muscle and bone may be involved

hematoma The collection of blood under the skin and tissues

incision An open wound with clean, straight edges; usually intentionally produced with a sharp instrument

infected wound A wound that contains large amounts of bacteria and that shows signs of infection; a dirty wound

intentional wound A wound created for therapy

laceration Open wound with torn tissues and jagged edges

open wound The skin or mucous membrane is broken

partial-thickness wound A wound in which the dermis and epidermis of the skin are broken

penetrating wound An open wound in which the skin and underlying tissues are pierced

puncture wound An open wound made by a sharp object; entry of the skin and underlying tissues may be intentional or unintentional

purulent drainage Thick, green, yellow, or brown drainage

sanguineous drainage Bloody drainage *(sanguis)*

serosanguineous drainage Thin, watery drainage *(sero)* that is blood-tinged *(sanguineous)*

serous drainage Clear, watery fluid *(serum)*

trauma An accident or violent act that injures the skin, mucous membranes, bones, and internal organs

unintentional wound A wound resulting from trauma

wound A break in the skin or mucous membrane

A wound is a break in the skin or mucous membrane. Wounds result from many causes. A surgical incision leaves a wound. Often wounds result from **trauma**—an accident or violent act that injures the skin, mucous membranes, bones, and internal organs. Falls, vehicle accidents, gun shots, stabbings, and other violent acts are sources of trauma. Human and animal bites, burns, and frostbite are other types of trauma. Pressure sores (pressure ulcers) are wounds that occur from poor skin care and immobility.

The wound is a portal of entry for microorganisms. Thus infection is a major threat. Wound care involves preventing infection and preventing further injury to the wound and surrounding tissues. Preventing blood loss and pain also are important.

Your role in wound care depends on state law, your job description, and the person's condition. Whatever your role, you need to know the types of wounds, how wounds heal, and the measures that promote wound healing. A review of surgical asepsis is useful before studying this chapter (see Chapter 2).

TYPES OF WOUNDS

Wounds are described in many ways. They are intentional or unintentional, open or closed, clean or dirty, and partial-thickness or full-thickness. **Intentional wounds** are created for therapy. Surgical incisions and venipunctures for starting IV therapy or for collecting blood specimens are examples. **Unintentional wounds** result from trauma. Falls, vehicle accidents, gun shots, stabbings, and other violent acts are sources of unintentional wounds.

A wound is open or closed. An **open wound** is when the skin or mucous membrane is broken. Intentional and most unintentional wounds are open. In a **closed wound,** tissues are injured but the skin is not broken. Bruises, twists, and sprains are examples of closed wounds.

Contamination is another factor in describing wounds. A **clean wound** is not infected, and microbes have not entered the wound. Closed wounds are usually clean. So are intentional wounds created under surgically aseptic conditions. In addition, the urinary, respiratory, and gastrointestinal systems are not entered. A **clean-contaminated wound** occurs from the surgical entry of the urinary, reproductive, respiratory, or gastrointestinal system. Except for the urinary system, these systems are not sterile and contain normal flora. A **contaminated wound** has a high risk of infection. Unintentional wounds are generally contaminated. Wound contamination also occurs from breaks in surgical asepsis and spillage of intestinal contents. Tissues may show signs of inflammation. An **infected wound** (**dirty wound**) contains large amounts of bacteria and shows signs of infection. Examples include old wounds, surgical incisions into infected areas, and traumatic injuries that rupture the bowel. A **chronic wound** is one that does not heal easily. Pressure sores and ulcers in persons with circulatory disorders are examples. (See Chapter 13 in *Mosby's Textbook for Nursing Assistants* (edition 4) for a review of pressure sores).

Partial or full thickness describes a wound's depth. In a **partial-thickness wound,** the dermis and epidermis of the skin are broken. The dermis, epidermis, and subcutaneous tissue are penetrated in a **full-thickness wound.** Muscle and bone may be involved.

Wounds are described also by their cause:

- **Abrasion**—a partial-thickness wound caused by the scraping away or rubbing of the skin
- **Contusion**—a closed wound caused by a blow to the body
- **Incision**—an open wound with clean, straight edges; usually intentionally produced with a sharp instrument
- **Laceration**—an open wound with torn tissues and jagged edges
- **Penetrating wound**—an open wound in which the skin and underlying tissues are pierced
- **Puncture wound**—an open wound made by a sharp object; entry of the skin and underlying tissues may be intentional or unintentional

WOUND HEALING

The healing process has three phases:

- *Inflammatory phase* (3 days)—Bleeding stops, and a scab forms over the wound. The scab protects microorganisms from entering the wound. Blood supply to the wound increases. The blood brings nutrients and healing substances. Because of the increased blood supply, signs and symptoms of inflammation appear: redness, swelling, heat or warmth, and pain. Loss of function may occur.
- *Proliferative phase* (day 3 to day 21)—Proliferate means to multiply rapidly. During this phase, tissue cells multiply to repair the wound.
- *Maturation phase* (day 21 to 1 or 2 years)—The scar gains strength. The red, raised scar eventually becomes thin and pale.

Types of Wound Healing

The healing process occurs through primary intention, secondary intention, or tertiary intention. With *primary intention (first intention, primary closure),* the wound edges are brought together. This closes the wound. Sutures (stitches), staples, clips, or adhesive strips hold the wound edges together. Special glues are now available to doctors for wound closings.

Secondary intention (second intention) is used for contaminated and infected wounds. Wounds are cleaned and dead tissue removed. Wound edges are not brought together, and the wound gaps. Healing occurs naturally. However, healing takes longer and leaves a larger scar. The threat of infection is great.

Tertiary intention (third intention, delayed intention) involves leaving a wound open and then closing it later. Thus tertiary intention combines secondary and primary intention. Infection and poor circulation are common reasons for tertiary intention.

Complications of Wound Healing

Many factors affect the healing process and increase the risk of complications. The type of wound is one factor. Other factors include the person's age, general health, nutrition, and life-style. Good circulation is important. Age, smoking, circulatory disease, and diabetes all affect circulation. Certain medications (Coumadin and heparin) can prolong bleeding. Tissue growth and repair require adequate protein in the diet. Infection is a risk for persons with immune system changes and for those taking antibiotics.

Hemorrhage *Hemorrhage* is the excessive loss of blood in a short period of time. If the bleeding is not stopped, death results. Hemorrhage may be internal or external. Internal hemorrhage cannot be seen. Bleeding occurs inside the body into tissues and body cavities. A **hematoma** may form. A hematoma is a collection of blood under the skin and tissues. The area appears swollen and has a reddish blue color. Shock, vomiting blood, coughing up blood, and loss of consciousness are signs of internal hemorrhage.

You can see external bleeding. Bloody drainage and dressings soaked with blood are common signs. Remember, gravity causes fluid to flow down. Therefore blood can flow down and collect under the part. Always check under the body part for the pooling of blood. As with internal hemorrhage, shock can occur.

Shock results when there is not enough blood supply to organs and tissues. Signs and symptoms include low or falling blood pressure, a rapid and weak pulse, and rapid respirations. The skin is cold, moist, and pale. The person is restless and may complain of thirst. Confusion and loss of consciousness occur as shock worsens.

Hemorrhage and shock are emergencies. Immediately notify the RN, and assist as requested. Remember to practice Standard Precautions and follow the Bloodborne Pathogen Standard when in contact with blood. Gloves are always worn. Gowns, masks, and eye protection are necessary when blood splashes and splatters are likely.

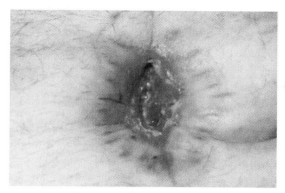

Fig. 3-1 *Wound dehiscence. (Courtesy Morison M:* A colour guide to the nursing management of wounds, *London, 1992, Mosby-Wolfe.)*

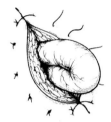

Fig. 3-2 *Wound evisceration. (From* Mosby's medical, nursing, & allied health dictionary, *ed 5, St Louis, 1998, Mosby.)*

Infection Wound contamination can occur during or after the injury. Trauma is a common source of contaminated wounds. Surgical wounds can be contaminated during or after surgery. An infected wound appears inflamed (reddened) and has drainage (p. 40). The wound is painful and tender. The person has a fever.

Dehiscence **Dehiscence** is the separation of the wound layers (Fig. 3-1). Separation may involve the skin layer or underlying tissues. Abdominal wounds are most commonly affected. Coughing, vomiting, and abdominal distention place stress on the wound. The person often describes the sensation of the wound popping open.

Evisceration **Evisceration** is the separation of the wound along with the protrusion of abdominal organs (Fig. 3-2). Causes are the same as for dehiscence.

Dehiscence and evisceration are surgical emergencies. The wound is covered with large sterile dressings saturated with sterile saline. You must notify the RN immediately and assist in preparing the person for surgery.

BOX 3-1 WOUND OBSERVATIONS

Wound location
- Multiple wounds may exist from surgery or trauma.

Wound size and depth (measure in centimeters)
- Size: measure from top to bottom and side to side.
- Depth (1) insert a sterile swab inside the deepest part of the wound; (2) remove the swab and measure the distance on the swab. *Measure depth only when the wound is open and with the RN's supervision.*
- Use the same ruler when measuring the wound.

Wound appearance
- Is the wound red and swollen?
- Is the area around the wound warm to touch?
- Are sutures, staples, or clips intact or broken?
- Are wound edges closed or separated? Did the wound break open?

Drainage (see p. 40)
- Is the drainage serous, sanguineous, serosanguineous, or purulent?
- What is the amount of drainage?

Odor
- Does the wound or drainage have an odor?

Surrounding skin
- Is surrounding skin intact?
- What is the color of surrounding skin?
- Are surrounding tissues swollen? ※

Wound Appearance

During the healing process, doctors and nurses routinely observe the wound and its drainage. They observe for healing and complications. You need to make certain observations when assisting with wound care. You report your observations to the RN and record them according to facility policy. Box 3-1 lists the wound observations that you need to make.

Wound Drainage

During injury and the inflammatory phase of wound healing, fluid and cells escape from the tissues. The amount of drainage may be small or large depending on wound size and location. Bleeding and infection also affect the amount and kind of drainage. Wound drainage is observed and measured.

Major types of wound drainage are as follows:

- **Serous drainage**—clear, watery fluid (Fig. 3-3, *A*). The fluid in a blister is serous. *Serous* comes from the word *serum*, which is the clean, thin, fluid portion of the blood. Serum does not contain blood cells or platelets.

- **Sanguineous drainage**—bloody drainage (Fig. 3-3, *B*). Sanguineous comes from the Latin word *sanguis*, which means blood. The amount and color of sanguineous drainage is important. Hemorrhage is suspected when large amounts are present. Bright drainage indicates fresh bleeding. Older bleeding is darker.

- **Serosanguineous drainage**—thin, watery drainage *(sero)* that is blood-tinged *(sanguineous)* (Fig. 3-3, *C*).

- **Purulent drainage**—thick drainage that is green, yellow, or brown (Fig. 3-3, *D*)

Drainage must leave the wound for healing to occur. If drainage is trapped inside the wound, underlying tissues swell. The wound may heal at the skin level, but underlying tissues do not close. This can lead to infection and other complications.

When large amounts of drainage are expected, the doctor inserts a drain. A *Penrose drain* is a rubber tube that drains onto a dressing (Fig. 3-4). Because the Penrose drain opens onto the dressing, it is an open drain and a portal of entry for microbes.

Closed drainage systems prevent microbes from entering the wound. A drainage tube is placed in the wound and attached to suction. The Hemovac (Fig. 3-5) and Jackson-Pratt (Fig. 3-6) systems are examples. Other systems are used depending on the type of wound, its size, and location.

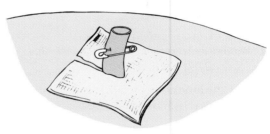

Fig. 3-4 *A Penrose drain. The safety pin prevents the drain from slipping into the wound. (From Potter PA, Perry AG:* Fundamentals of nursing: concepts, process, and practice, *ed 4, St Louis, 1997, Mosby.)*

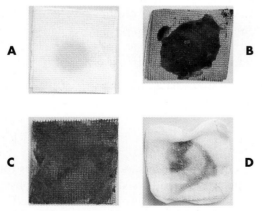

Fig. 3-3 *Wound drainage.* **A,** *Serous drainage.* **B,** *Sanguineous drainage.* **C,** *Serosanguineous drainage.* **D,** *Purulent drainage.* *(From Potter PA, Perry AG:* Fundamentals of nursing: concepts, process, and practice, *ed 4, St Louis, 1997, Mosby.)*

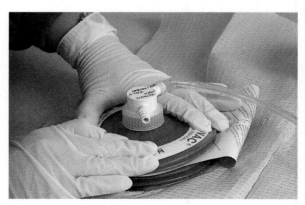

Fig. 3-5 *A Hemovac. Drains are sutured to the wound and connected to the reservoir. (From Elkin MK, Perry AG, Potter PA:* Nursing interventions and clinical skills, *1996, Mosby.)*

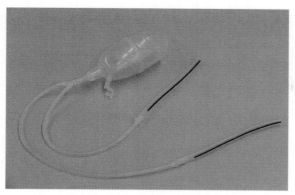

Fig. 3-6 *The Jackson-Pratt drainage system. (From Elkin MK, Perry AG, Potter PA: Nursing interventions and clinical skills, 1996, Mosby.)*

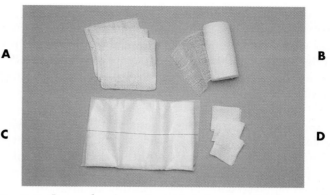

Fig. 3-7 *Gauze dressings.* **A,** *4 × 4 dressing.* **B,** *Gauze roll.* **C,** *Abdominal pad (ABD).* **D,** *2 × 2 dressing.*

Drainage is measured in three ways:

- Note the number and size of dressings with drainage. Describe the amount and kind of drainage on them. Are dressings saturated? Is drainage on just part of the dressing? If so, which part? Is drainage through some or all layers of the dressing?

- Weigh dressings before applying them to the wound. Note the weight of each dressing. Note the weight of each dressing after removal. Subtract the weight of the dry dressing from the wet dressing.

- Measure the amount of drainage in the collecting receptacle if closed drainage is used.

DRESSINGS

Wound dressings have many functions. They protect wounds from injury and microbes. Drainage is absorbed and removed along with dead tissue. Dressings can promote comfort and cover unsightly wounds. They also provide a moist environment for wound healing. When bleeding is a problem, pressure dressings help control bleeding.

The type and size of dressing used depends on many factors. These include the type of wound, its size, and location; amount of drainage; and the presence or absence of infection. The dressing's function and the frequency of dressing changes are other factors. The RN tells you what dressing to use.

Types of Dressings

Dressings are described by the material used and application method. Many products are available for dressing wounds. You need to be familiar with the following materials:

- *Gauze*—comes in squares, rectangles, pads, and rolls (Fig. 3-7). Gauze dressings absorb moisture.

- *Nonadherent gauze*—is a gauze dressing with a non-stick surface. The dressing does not stick to the wound and removes easily without injuring tissue.

- *Transparent adhesive film*—prevent fluids and bacteria from reaching the wound, but air can. The wound is kept moist. Drainage is not absorbed. The transparent film allows wound observation.

Some dressings contain special agents to promote wound healing. The RN is likely to change such dressings. If you assist with the dressing change, the RN explains its use to you.

Dressing application methods involve dry and wet dressings:

- *Dry-to-dry dressing* (usually called a *dry dressing*)—A dry gauze dressing is placed over the wound. Additional dressings are placed on top of the first dressing as needed. Drainage is absorbed by the dressing and is removed with the dressing. A dry dressing can stick to the wound. The dressing must be removed carefully to prevent tissue injury and discomfort.

- *Wet-to-dry dressing*—A gauze dressing saturated with a solution is applied over the wound. Additional dressings are applied as needed. These dressings are also moistened with solution. The solution softens dead tissue in the wound. The dead tissue is absorbed by the dressing and is removed with the dressing. The dressings are removed when dry.

- *Wet-to-wet dressing*—Gauze dressings saturated with solution are placed in the wound. The dressing is kept moist.

Securing Dressings

Dressings must be secure over wounds. Bacteria can enter the wound and drainage can escape if the dressing is dislodged. Tape and Montgomery ties are commonly used to secure dressings. Binders (pp. 45-46) also hold dressings in place.

Tape Adhesive, paper, plastic, and elastic tapes are available. Adhesive tape sticks well to the skin. However, the adhesive part can remain on the skin and is hard to remove. The adhesive can irritate the skin. Sometimes skin is removed with the tape, causing an abrasion. Many people are allergic to adhesive tape. Paper and plastic tapes are nonallergenic. This means that they do not cause allergic reactions. Elastic tape allows movement of the body part. The RN tells you what type of tape to use for the person.

Tape is available in ½-inch, 1-inch, 2-inch, and 3-inch widths. The size used depends on the size of the dressing. The RN tells you what size to use. Tape is applied to secure the top, middle, and bottom of the dressing (Fig. 3-8). The tape should extend beyond each side of the dressing. *The tape should not encircle the entire body part. If swelling occurs, circulation to the part is impaired.*

Montgomery ties Montgomery ties (Fig. 3-9) are used for large dressings and when frequent dressing changes are needed. A Montgomery tie consists of an adhesive strip and a cloth tie. When the dressing is in place, the adhesive strips are placed on both sides of the dressing. Then the cloth ties are secured over the dressing. Two or three Montgomery ties may be needed on each side. The cloth ties are undone for the dressing change. The adhesive strips are not removed unless soiled.

focus on children Children are often afraid of dressing changes. Tape removal is often painful for them. The wound's appearance can be frightening. A calm, cooperative child is important to prevent contamination of the sterile field. Let the parent or caregiver hold the child if you can reach the wound with ease. Letting the child hold or play with a favorite toy is often comforting.

focus on older persons Older persons have thin, fragile skin. You must prevent skin tears. Extreme care is necessary when removing tape.

focus on home care Make sure you have the necessary supplies before leaving the agency. The RN may ask you to telephone him or her after removing the old dressings. During this telephone call, you report your observations to the RN. Then the RN gives you instructions about how to proceed.

Applying Dressings

The doctor usually does the first dressing change after surgery. The RN follows the doctor's order for dressing changes. The RN tells you when to change a dressing and what supplies to use. A dressing change usually involves cleaning the wound and drain site. Box 3-2 lists the rules for applying dressings. Box 3-3 lists the rules for cleaning wounds and drain sites.

Remember, assistive personnel do not administer medications. The doctor's orders may include applying a medicated powder or ointment to the wound. The RN is responsible for applying the medication. Also, some wounds and dressings are more complex than others. An RN observes such wounds and changes the dressings. Your job description may allow you to apply simple dressings to uncomplicated wounds and to assist the RN with complex wounds.

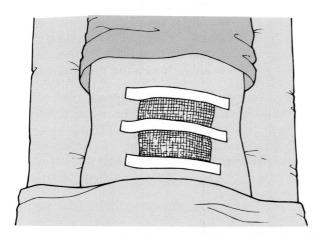

Fig. 3-8 *Tape is applied at the top, middle, and bottom of the dressing. Note that the tape extends beyond both sides of the dressing.*

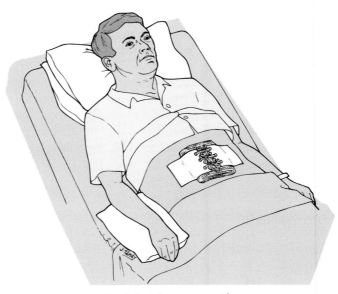

Fig. 3-9 *Montgomery ties.*

BOX 3-2 RULES FOR APPLYING DRESSINGS

- Make sure your state allows assistive personnel to perform the procedure.
- Make sure the procedure is in your job description.
- Apply dressings only under the RN's direction and supervision.
- Review the procedure with the RN. A patient may require special measures.
- Allow pain medications time to take effect. The person may experience discomfort during the dressing change. The RN gives the medication and tells you how long to wait.
- Provide for the person's fluid and elimination needs before starting the procedure.
- Collect all needed equipment and supplies before you begin.
- Control your nonverbal communication. Wound odors, appearance, and drainage may be unpleasant. Do not communicate your thoughts and reactions to the person.
- Remove soiled dressings so that the underside of the dressing is away from the person's sight. The drainage and its odor may upset the person.
- Do not force the person to look at the wound. A wound can affect the person's body image and esteem. The RN helps the person deal with the wound.
- Practice Standard Precautions, and follow the Bloodborne Pathogen Standard. Wear personal protective equipment as necessary.
- Wear clean, disposable gloves to remove old dressings.
- Remove tape by pulling the tape toward the wound.
- Remove dressings gently to prevent pain and discomfort. The dressing may stick to the wound and surrounding skin.
- Follow the rules of surgical asepsis to apply a sterile dressing (see p. 24).
- Set up your sterile field after removing and discarding old dressings.
- Wear sterile gloves to apply new dressings.
- Follow the rules for cleaning wounds and drain sites (see Box 3-3). ✳

BOX 3-3 RULES FOR CLEANING WOUNDS AND DRAIN SITES

- Ask the RN about what solution to use.
- Use sterile gauze dressings to apply the solution.
- Use sterile forceps to hold the sterile gauze for cleaning.
- Clean away from the wound. Clean fro44m the wound to the surrounding skin (Fig. 3-10).
- Use circular motions when cleaning drain sites (Fig. 3-11).
- Use a different gauze dressing for each stroke. ✳

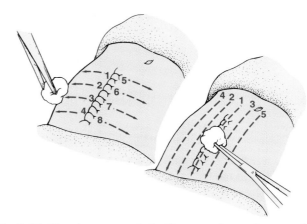

Fig. 3-10 *Cleaning a wound.* **A,** *Clean starting at the wound and stroking out to surrounding skin.* **B,** *Clean the wound from top to bottom. Start at the wound. Then clean surrounding tissues. Remember to use a new swab for each stroke.* (From Potter PA, Perry AG: Fundamentals of nursing: concepts, process, and practice, ed 4, St Louis, 1997, Mosby.)

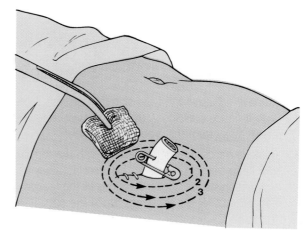

Fig. 3-11 *Cleaning a drain site. Clean in circular motions starting at the drain site. Use a new swab for each stroke.*

APPLYING A DRY STERILE DRESSING

PRE-PROCEDURE

1 Review the procedure with the RN.

2 Explain to the person what you are going to do.

3 Allow time for pain medication to take effect.

4 Provide for the person's fluid and elimination needs.

5 Wash your hands.

6 Collect needed equipment:
- Disposable gloves
- Sterile gloves
- Personal protective equipment as needed (mask, gown, eye shield)
- Sterile cleaning solution
- Sterile dressing set with sterile scissors and sterile forceps
- Sterile basin
- Sterile drape
- Tape and Montgomery ties as directed by the RN
- Sterile dressings as directed by the RN
- Sterile gauze swabs for wound cleaning
- Adhesive remover
- Leakproof bag
- Bath blanket

7 Identify the person. Check the ID bracelet with the assignment sheet. Provide for privacy.

8 Arrange furniture for your work surface. Make sure that you will not have to reach over or turn your back on the work surface.

9 Raise the bed to a level for good body mechanics. Make sure the far bed rail is raised.

PROCEDURE

10 Help the person to a comfortable position.

11 Cover the person with a bath blanket. Fanfold top linens to the foot of the bed.

12 Expose the affected body part.

13 Remind the person not to touch supplies or the wound.

14 Make a cuff on the leakproof bag. Place the bag within easy reach.

15 Put on the clean gown and mask if needed.

16 Put on the disposable gloves.

17 Undo Montgomery ties or remove tape:

   a Montgomery ties: fold ties away from the wound.

   b Tape: Hold the skin down, and gently pull the tape toward the wound.

18 Remove adhesive from the skin if necessary. Wet a 4×4 gauze dressing with the adhesive remover. Clean away from the wound.

19 Remove gauze dressings starting with the top dressing. Keep the soiled side of the dressing away from the person's sight. Place dressings in the leakproof bag. Do not let the dressings touch the outside of the bag.

20 Remove the dressing directly over the wound very gently. The dressing may stick to the wound or drain.

21 Observe the wound, drain site, and wound drainage (see Box 3-1).

22 Remove the disposable gloves. Discard them into the leakproof bag.

23 Make sure the leakproof bag is away from where you will set up your sterile field.

24 Wash your hands. Raise the side rail when you leave the bedside, and lower it upon your return.

25 Set up your sterile field (see Chapter 2):

   a Place the sterile drape over your work surface.

   b Open the sterile dressing set. Drop the contents onto the sterile field.

   c Open the sterile dressings. Drop them onto the sterile field.

   d Open the sterile bowl. Place it on the sterile field.

   e Open the sterile swabs for cleaning the wound. Drop them into the sterile bowl.

   f Open the sterile cleaning solution. Pour the solution into the bowl with the sterile swabs. Place the cap and bottle outside the sterile field.

APPLYING A DRY STERILE DRESSING—CONT'D

PROCEDURE—CONT'D

26 Put on the sterile gloves.

27 Pick up the sterile swabs with the sterile forceps. Place them in the cleaning solution. Save some swabs for drying the skin around the wound and drain site.

28 Clean the wound (see Fig. 3-10). Clean from the wound outward. Use a new swab for each stroke. Drop used swabs into the leakproof bag. Do not let the forceps touch the bag.

29 Clean around the drain site (see Fig. 3-11). Clean from the wound outward. Use a new swab for each circular motion. Do not let the forceps touch the bag.

30 Dry the skin around the wound and drain site. Use dry swabs.

31 Apply a 4 × 4 gauze dressing to the drain site (see Fig. 3-4). Use a precut 4 × 4 dressing, or cut halfway through a 4 × 4 dressing using the sterile scissors.

32 Apply dressings over the wound and drain site as directed by the RN.

33 Secure the dressings in place. Use tape (see Fig. 3-8) or Montgomery ties (see Fig. 3-9).

34 Remove your gloves. Discard them in the leakproof bag.

POST-PROCEDURE

35 Help the person to assume a comfortable position. Cover the person with the top linens, and remove the bath blanket.

36 Make sure the call bell is within the person's reach.

37 Lower the bed to its lowest position. Raise or lower side rails as instructed by the RN.

38 Unscreen the person.

39 Discard supplies into the leakproof bag. Discard the leakproof bag according to facility policy.

40 Clean your work surface following the Bloodborne Pathogen Standard. Return furniture to its proper place.

41 Wash your hands.

42 Report your observations to the RN.

BINDERS

Binders are applied to the abdomen, chest, or perineal areas. Binders promote healing because they:

- Support wounds and hold dressings in place
- Reduce or prevent swelling by promoting circulation
- Promote comfort
- Prevent injury

Binders must be applied properly. Incorrect application can cause severe discomfort, skin irritation, and circulatory and respiratory complications. The binder's effectiveness and the person's safety depend on correct application. Box 3-4 on p. 46 lists the rules for applying these binders:

- *Straight abdominal binders*—provide abdominal support and hold dressings in place (Fig. 3-12, p. 46). The binder is a rectangle. The binder is applied with the person supine. The top part is positioned at the person's waist. The lower part is over the hips. The binder is secured in place with pins, hooks, or Velcro.

- *Breast binders*—support the breasts following breast surgery (Fig. 3-13, p. 46). They also apply pressure to the breasts after childbirth. If the mother does not breast-feed, pressure from the binder helps dry up the milk in the breasts. The binder also promotes comfort and provides support to swollen breasts after childbirth. The woman is supine when the breast binder is applied. The binder is pulled snugly across the chest and secured in place.

- *T binders*—used to secure dressings in place after rectal and perineal surgeries. The single T binder is used for women (Fig. 3-14, *A*, p. 46). The double T binder is used for men (Fig. 3-14, *B*, p. 46). If perineal dressings are large, women may need double T binders. To apply a T binder, the waist bands are brought around the waist and pinned at the front. The tails are brought between the person's legs and up to the waistband. They are pinned in place at the waistband.

BOX 3-4 RULES FOR APPLYING BINDERS

- Apply the binder so that firm, even pressure is exerted over the area.
- Apply the binder so it is snug but does not interfere with breathing or circulation.
- Position the person in good alignment when the binder is applied.

- Reapply the binder if it becomes loose, wrinkled, or out of position or causes discomfort.
- Secure pins so they point away from incisional areas.
- Change binders that are moist or soiled to prevent the growth of microorganisms. ※

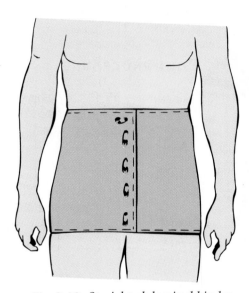

Fig. 3-12 *Straight abdominal binder.*

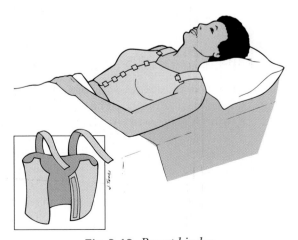

Fig. 3-13 *Breast binder.*

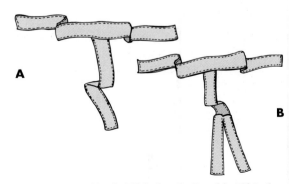

Fig. 3-14 **A,** *Single T binder.* **B,** *Double T binder.*

HEAT AND COLD APPLICATIONS

Heat and cold applications are often ordered for wound care. Heat and cold applications are ordered by doctors to promote healing, promote comfort, and reduce tissue swelling. Refer to Chapter 23 in *Mosby's Textbook for Nursing Assistants* (edition 4) for a review of heat and cold applications.

WOUND CARE AND THE PERSON'S BASIC NEEDS

This chapter focuses on wounds. However, you must remember that it is the *person* who has the wound. The wound, which can affect the person's basic needs, is only one aspect of the person's care.

You must remember that the person is recovering from surgery or trauma. The wound is a source of pain and discomfort. The wound and the pain may interfere with breathing and moving. Turning, repositioning, and ambulating may be painful. You must handle the person gently and allow pain medications to take effect before giving care.

Good nutrition is needed for healing. However, pain and discomfort can affect the person's appetite. So can odors from wound drainage. Remove soiled dressings promptly from the room, use room deodorizers, and keep drainage containers out of the person's sight. If the person has a taste for certain foods or beverages, report this information to the RN.

Infection is always a threat. You must practice Standard Precautions and follow the Bloodborne Pathogen Standard. Dressing changes require sterile technique. Also, observe the wound and the person carefully for signs and symptoms of infection.

Delayed healing is a risk for persons who are elderly or obese or have poor nutrition. Poor circulation and diabetes also affect healing. These conditions are risk factors for infection.

Many fears affect the person's sense of safety and security. The person fears scarring, disfigurement, delayed healing, and infection. Fears about the wound "popping" open are common. Costly medical bills are other concerns. Continued hospital care, home care, or long-term care may be needed.

Victims of violence have many other concerns. Future attacks, finding and convicting the attacker, and fear for family members are common concerns. Victims of domestic violence, child abuse, and elderly abuse often hide the true source of their injuries.

The person's wound may be large or small. It may be visible to others—on the face, arms, or legs—or hidden by clothing. Wound drainage may have unpleasant odors. The wound may be extensive and disfiguring. It may affect the person's ability to perform sexually or the person's sense of being sexually attractive. The amputation of a finger, hand, arm, toe, foot, or leg can affect the person's function, everyday activities, and job. Eye injuries can affect vision. Abdominal trauma and surgery can affect eating and elimination.

Whatever the location or size of the wound, physical function and body image are affected. The person's sense of love and belonging and self-esteem are affected. You must be sensitive to the person's feelings. The person may be sad and tearful or angry and hostile. Adjustment may be difficult and rehabilitation necessary. You must be gentle and kind, give thoughtful care, and practice good communication techniques. Other health team members—social workers, psychiatrists, and the clergy—may be involved in the person's care.

SUMMARY

Assisting with wound care is an important function. A wound provides a portal of entry for microbes. Preventing infection is important. You must protect the person and yourself from infection. Standard Precautions, surgical asepsis, and the Bloodborne Pathogen Standard are followed.

Infection, hemorrhage, shock, and wound dehiscence and evisceration are possible wound complications. You assist the RN in preventing these complications through alert and careful observation of the person and the wound. Report signs and symptoms of complications to the RN immediately.

You must follow the RN's directions when assisting with wound care. Make sure you understand what the RN wants you to do. You must be comfortable with the procedure and required supplies and equipment before going to the patient.

The wound can affect the person's basic needs. Physical, safety and security, love and belonging, and self-esteem needs are affected. Wound size and site can affect the person's activities of daily living, work, and play. You must be sensitive to how the wound affects the person.

REVIEW QUESTIONS

Circle the best *answer.*

1 Sally Jones fell off her bike. She has a laceration on her right leg. Which is *false?*
a She has an open wound.
b She has an infected wound.
c She has a contaminated wound.
d She has an unintentional wound.

2 A person had rectal surgery. What type of wound does the person have?
a A clean wound
b A dirty wound
c A clean-contaminated wound
d A contaminated wound

3 The skin and underlying tissues are pierced. This is
a A penetrating wound
b An incision
c A contusion
d An abrasion

4 A wound appears red and swollen. The area around the wound is warm to touch. These signs are characteristics of
a The inflammatory phase of wound healing
b The proliferative phase of wound healing
c Healing by primary intention
d Healing by secondary intention

5 A wound is healing by primary intention. During a dressing change you note that the wound is separating. This is called
a Dehiscence
b Tertiary intention
c Evisceration
d Hematoma

6 You note a clear, watery drainage from a wound. This drainage is called
a Purulent drainage
b Serous drainage
c Seropurulent drainage
d Serosanguineous drainage

7 You note large amounts of sanguineous drainage in a Hemovac. Which is *true?*
a The person is bleeding.
b You need to notify the doctor.
c The person has an infection.
d The person has a Penrose drain.

8 A dressing does the following *except*
a Protect the wound from injury
b Absorb drainage
c Provide a moist environment for wound healing
d Support the wound and reduce swelling

9 Which dressing is likely to stick to a wound?
a A wet-to-wet dressing
b Nonadherent gauze
c A dry-to-dry dressing
d Montgomery ties

10 You are securing a dressing with tape. Tape is applied
a Around the entire part
b To the top and bottom of the dressing
c To the top, middle, and bottom of the dressing
d As the person prefers

11 You are going to apply a sterile dressing. You put on sterile gloves
a At the beginning of the procedure
b To remove the old dressings
c To open sterile dressings
d After setting up the sterile field

REVIEW QUESTIONS—CONT'D

12 When cleaning a wound, you clean
   a Outward from the wound
   b Toward the wound
   c In circular motions away from the wound
   d In circular motions toward the wound

13 The wound is cleaned
   a After setting up the sterile field
   b While wearing clean disposable gloves
   c With soap and water
   d Daily

14 Mr. Moore has an abdominal binder. The binder is used to
   a Prevent blood clots
   b Prevent wound infection
   c Provide support and hold dressings in place
   d Decrease circulation and swelling

Answers to these questions are on p. 179

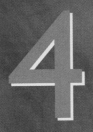

4 *Assisting With Oxygen Needs*

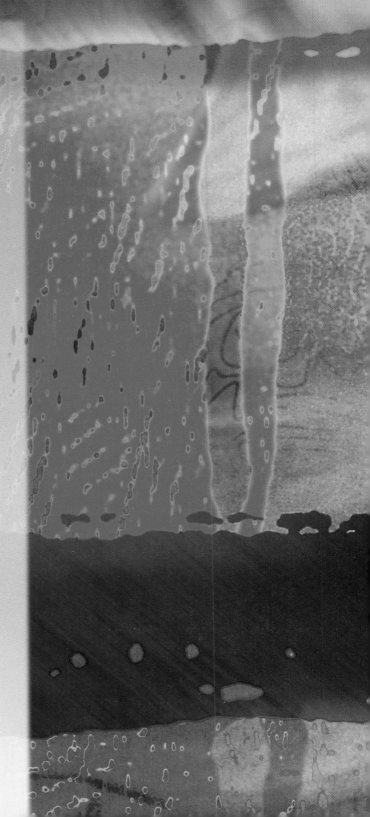

OBJECTIVES

- Define key terms
- Describe the factors affecting oxygen needs
- Identify the signs and symptoms of hypoxia and altered respiratory function
- Describe the tests used to diagnose respiratory problems
- Explain how positioning, coughing and deep breathing, and incentive spirometry promote oxygenation
- Describe the devices used to administer oxygen
- Explain how to safely assist with oxygen therapy
- Explain how to assist in the care of persons with artificial airways
- Describe the safety measures for oral suctioning
- Explain how to assist in the care of persons on mechanical ventilation
- Explain how to assist in the care of persons with chest tubes
- Perform the procedures described in this chapter

KEY TERMS

allergy A sensitivity to a substance that causes the body to react with signs and symptoms

apnea The lack or absence *(a)* of breathing *(pnea)*

Biot's respirations Irregular breathing with periods of apnea; respirations may be slow and deep or rapid and shallow

bradypnea Slow *(brady)* breathing *(pnea)*; respirations are fewer than 10 per minute

Cheyne-Stokes Respirations gradually increase in rate and depth and then become shallow and slow; breathing may stop *(apnea)* for 10 to 20 seconds

dyspnea Difficult, labored, or painful *(dys)* breathing *(pnea)*

hemoptysis Bloody *(hemo)* sputum *(ptysis* meaning "to spit")

hemothorax The collection of blood *(hemo)* in the pleural space *(thorax)*

hyperventilation Respirations that are rapid *(hyper)* and deeper than normal

hypoventilation Respirations that are slow *(hypo)*, shallow, and sometimes irregular

hypoxemia A reduced amount *(hypo)* of oxygen *(ox)* in the blood *(emia)*

hypoxia A deficiency *(hypo)* of oxygen in the cells *(oxia)*

Kussmaul's respirations Very deep and rapid respirations; a sign of diabetic coma

orthopnea Being able to breathe *(pnea)* deeply and comfortably only while sitting or standing *(ortho)*

orthopneic position Sitting up in bed *(ortho)* and leaning forward over the bedside table

oxygen concentration The amount of hemoglobin that contains oxygen (O_2)

pleural effusion The escape and collection of fluid *(effusion)* in the pleural space

pneumothorax The collection of air *(pneumo)* in the pleural space *(thorax)*

pollutant A harmful chemical or substance in the air or water

respiratory arrest Breathing stops

respiratory depression Slow, weak respirations that occur at a rate of fewer than 12 per minute; respirations are not deep enough to bring enough air into the lungs

sputum Expectorated mucus

suction The process of withdrawing or sucking up fluid *(secretions)*

tachypnea Rapid *(tachy)* breathing *(pnea)*; respirations are usually more than 24 per minute

Oxygen (O_2) is a tasteless, odorless, and colorless gas. It is a basic need—necessary for survival. Death occurs within minutes if a person stops breathing. Serious illnesses occur without enough oxygen. Illness, surgery, and injuries affect the amount of oxygen in the blood and cells.

FACTORS AFFECTING OXYGEN NEEDS

The respiratory and cardiovascular systems must function properly for cells to get enough oxygen. Any disease, injury, or surgery involving these systems affects the body's ability to take in oxygen and deliver it to the cells. Each body system depends on the other. Altered function of any system (for example, the nervous, musculoskeletal, or urinary system) affects the body's ability to meet its oxygen needs. Major factors affecting oxygen needs are:

- *Respiratory system status*—Structures must be intact and functioning. The airway must be open (patent). Alveoli must exchange O_2 and carbon dioxide (CO_2).

- *Cardiovascular system function*—Blood must flow freely to and from the heart. Narrowed vessels affect the delivery of oxygen-rich blood to the cells and blood return to the heart. Capillaries and cells must exchange O_2 and CO_2.

- *Red blood cell count*—The blood must have enough red blood cells (RBCs). RBCs contain hemoglobin, which picks up oxygen in the lungs and carries it to the cells. The bone marrow must produce enough RBCs. Poor diet, chemotherapy, and leukemia affect bone marrow function. Blood loss also reduces the number of RBCs.

- *Intact nervous system*—Nervous system diseases and injuries can affect respiratory muscle function. Breathing may be difficult or impossible. Brain damage affects respiratory rate, rhythm, and depth. Narcotics and depressant drugs are chemicals that affect the brain. They slow respirations. The amount of O_2 and CO_2 in the blood also affects brain function. Respirations increase when O_2 is lacking. The body tries to bring in more oxygen. Respirations also increase when CO_2 increases. The body tries to get rid of CO_2.

- *Aging*—Respiratory muscles weaken, and lung tissue becomes less elastic. There is decreased strength for coughing. Coughing and removing secretions from the upper airway are important. Otherwise, upper respiratory tract infections can lead to *pneumonia* (inflammation of the lung). Respiratory complications are a risk after surgery.

- *Exercise*—Oxygen needs increase with exercise. Normally, respiratory rate and depth increase to bring enough O_2 into the lungs. Persons with heart and respiratory diseases may have enough oxygen at rest. However, even slight activity can increase their oxygen needs. Their bodies may not be able to bring in oxygen and to deliver it to cells.

- *Fever*—Oxygen needs increase. As with exercise, respiratory rate and depth must increase to meet the body's needs.

- *Pain*—Pain increases the need for oxygen. Respirations increase to meet this need. However, chest and abdominal injuries and surgeries often involve the respiratory muscles. This interferes with breathing in and out.

- *Medications*—Some drugs depress the respiratory center in the brain. **Respiratory depression** is slow, weak respirations at a rate of fewer than 12 per minute. Respirations are too shallow to bring enough air into the lungs. **Respiratory arrest** is when breathing stops. Narcotics such as morphine and Demerol can have these effects. (The word *narcotic* comes from the Greek word *narkoun;* it means stupor or to be numb.) These drugs are given in safe amounts for severe pain. Substance abusers are at risk for respiratory depression and respiratory arrest from overdoses of narcotics and depressants. Narcotics include opium, heroin, and methadone. Depressant drugs include barbiturates (Nembutal, phenobarbital, secobarbital, Tuinal, and others) and the benzodiazepines (Dalmane, diazepam, Halcion, Librium, Tranxene, Valium, Xanax, and others).

- *Smoking*—Smoking causes lung cancer and chronic obstructive pulmonary disease (COPD). It is a risk factor for coronary artery disease.

- *Allergies*—An **allergy** is a sensitivity to a substance that causes the body to react with signs and symptoms. Respiratory signs and symptoms include runny nose, wheezing, and congestion. Mucous membranes in the upper airway swell. With severe swelling, the airway closes. Shock and death are risks. Pollens, dust, foods, drugs, and cigarette smoke often cause allergies. Persons with allergies are at risk for chronic bronchitis and asthma.

- *Pollutant exposure*—A **pollutant** is a harmful chemical or substance in the air or water. Dust, fumes, toxins, asbestos, coal dust, and sawdust are some air pollutants. They damage the lungs. Pollutant exposure occurs in home, work, and community settings.

- *Nutrition*—Good nutrition is needed for red blood cell production. RBCs live about 3 or 4 months. New ones must replace those that die off. The body needs iron and vitamins (vitamin B_{12}, vitamin C, and folic acid) to produce RBCs.

- *Substance abuse*—Alcohol depresses the brain. Excessive amounts reduce the cough reflex and increase the risk of aspiration. Obstructed airway and pneumonia are risks from aspiration. Respiratory depression and respiratory arrest are risks when narcotics and depressant drugs are abused.

ALTERED RESPIRATORY FUNCTION

Respiratory system function involves three processes. Air moves into and out of the lungs. Oxygen and carbon dioxide are exchanged at the alveoli. The blood transports O_2 to the cells and removes CO_2 from them. Respiratory function is altered if even one process is affected.

Hypoxia

Hypoxia is a deficiency *(hypo)* of oxygen in the cells *(oxia)*. Cells do not receive enough oxygen. Therefore they do not function properly. Hypoxia is caused by any illness, disease, injury, or surgery affecting respiratory function. The brain is very sensitive to inadequate oxygen. Restlessness is an early sign of hypoxia. So are dizziness and disorientation. Report signs and symptoms of hypoxia to the RN immediately (Box 4-1).

Hypoxia is life-threatening. The heart, brain, and other organs must receive enough oxygen to function. Oxygen is given, and treatment is directed at the cause of the hypoxia.

Abnormal Respirations

Normal respirations occur between 12 and 20 times per minute in the adult. Infants and children have faster rates. Respirations are normally quiet, effortless, and regular. Both sides of the chest rise and fall equally. The following breathing patterns are abnormal.

- **Tachypnea**—rapid *(tachy)* breathing *(pnea)*. Respirations are usually more than 24 per minute. Fever, exercise, pain, pregnancy, airway obstruction, and hypoxemia are common causes. **Hypoxemia** is a reduced amount *(hypo)* of oxygen *(ox)* in the blood *(emia)*.

- **Bradypnea**—slow *(brady)* breathing *(pnea)*. Respirations are fewer than 10 per minute. Bradypnea is seen with drug overdoses and central nervous system disorders.

BOX 4-1 SIGNS AND SYMPTOMS OF HYPOXIA

- Restlessness
- Dizziness
- Disorientation
- Confusion
- Behavior and personality changes
- Difficulty concentrating and following directions
- Apprehension
- Anxiety

- Fatigue
- Agitation
- Increased pulse rate
- Increased rate and depth of respirations
- Sitting position, often leaning forward
- Cyanosis (bluish color to the skin, lips, mucous membranes, and nail beds)
- Dyspnea ✳

- **Apnea**—the lack or absence *(a)* of breathing *(pnea)*. It occurs in cardiac arrest and respiratory arrest. Sleep apnea and periodic apnea of newborns are other types of apnea.

- **Hypoventilation**—respirations that are slow *(hypo)*, shallow, and sometimes irregular. Lung disorders affecting the alveoli are common causes. Pneumonia is an example. Other causes include obesity, airway obstruction, drug side effects, and nervous system and musculoskeletal disorders affecting the respiratory muscles.

- **Hyperventilation**—respirations that are rapid *(hyper)* and deeper than normal. Its many causes include asthma, emphysema, infection, fever, central nervous system disorders, hypoxia, anxiety, pain, and some drugs.

- **Dyspnea**—difficult, labored, or painful *(dys)* breathing *(pnea)*. Heart disease, exercise, and anxiety are common causes.

- **Cheyne-Stokes**—respirations gradually increase in rate and depth and then become shallow and slow. Breathing may stop (apnea) for 10 to 20 seconds. Drug overdose, heart failure, renal failure, and brain disorders are common causes. These respirations are common when death is near.

- **Orthopnea**—breathing *(pnea)* deeply and comfortably only while sitting or standing *(ortho)*. Common causes include emphysema, asthma, pneumonia, angina pectoris, and other heart and respiratory disorders.

- **Biot's respirations**—irregular breathing with periods of apnea. Respirations are slow and deep or rapid and shallow. They occur with central nervous system disorders.

- **Kussmaul's respirations**—very deep and rapid respirations. They are a sign of diabetic coma.

Assisting With Assessment and Diagnostic Testing

Altered respiratory function may be an acute or chronic problem. Doctors and nurses are always alert for altered respiratory function. Report your observations to the RN promptly and accurately (Box 4-2, p. 54). Quick action is necessary to meet the person's oxygen needs. Measures are taken to correct the situation and prevent the problem from getting worse.

The doctor orders tests to determine the cause of altered respiratory function. The following tests are common. You are likely to assist with pulse oximetry and in collecting sputum specimens:

- *Chest x-ray (CXR)*—An x-ray is taken of the chest. It is used to evaluate changes in the lungs. All clothing and jewelry from the waist to the neck are removed. The person wears a hospital gown.

- *Lung scan*—The lungs are scanned to see what areas are not getting air or blood. The person inhales radioactive gas and is injected with a radioisotope. *Radioactive* means to give off radiation. A *radioisotope* is an element that gives off radiation. Lung tissue getting air and blood flow "take up" the radioactive substances. A scanner senses areas with radioactive substances. As when having a chest x-ray, the person removes all clothing and jewelry from the waist to the neck. A hospital gown is worn.

BOX 4-2 SIGNS AND SYMPTOMS OF ALTERED RESPIRATORY FUNCTION

- Signs and symptoms of hypoxia (see Box 4-1)
- Any abnormal breathing pattern (see pp. 52-53)
- Complaints of shortness of breath or being "winded" or "short-winded"
- Cough (note frequency and time of day)
  * Dry and hacking
  * Harsh and barking
  * Productive (produces sputum) or nonproductive
- Sputum
  * Color—clear, white, yellow, green, brown, or red
  * Odor—none or foul odor
  * Consistency—thick, watery, or frothy (with bubbles or foam)
  * **Hemoptysis**—bloody *(hemo)* sputum *(ptysis* meaning "to spit"); note if the sputum is bright red, dark red, blood-tinged, or streaked with blood

- Noisy respirations
  * Wheezing
  * Wet sounding respirations
  * Crowing sounds
- Chest pain (note location)
  * Constant
  * Person's description (stabbing, knife-like, aching)
  * What makes it worse (movement, coughing, yawning, sneezing, sighing, deep breathing)
- Cyanosis
  * Skin
  * Mucous membranes
  * Lips
  * Nail beds
- Changes in vital signs
- Body position
  * Sitting upright
  * Leaning foward or hunched over a table ✳

- *Bronchoscopy*—A scope *(scopy)* is passed into the trachea and bronchi *(broncho)*. The doctor inspects the larynx, trachea, and bronchi for bleeding and tumors. The doctor can take tissue samples (biopsy) or remove mucous plugs and foreign objects. The person is NPO 6 to 8 hours before the procedure. This reduces the danger of vomiting and aspiration. A local or general anesthetic is given. After the procedure, the person is NPO and watched carefully until the gag and swallow reflexes return. They usually return in about 2 hours. Preoperative and postoperative care is given as directed by the RN.

- *Thoracentesis*—The pleura *(thora)* is punctured, and air or fluid is aspirated *(centesis)* from it. The doctor inserts a needle through the chest wall into the pleural sac. Injury or disease can cause the pleural sac to fill with air, blood, or fluid. This affects respiratory function. The procedure also is done to remove fluid for laboratory study or to inject anticancer drugs into the pleural sac. The procedure takes a few minutes. Vital signs are taken before a local anesthetic is given. The person sits up or leans forward and is asked not to talk, cough, or move suddenly (Fig. 4-1). Post-procedure care involves applying a dressing to the puncture site and taking vital signs. A chest x-ray is taken to check for lung damage. The person is checked often for shortness of breath, dyspnea, cough, sputum, chest pain, cyanosis, vital sign changes, and other respiratory signs and symptoms.

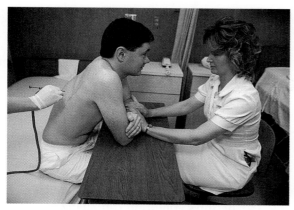

Fig. 4-1 *The person is positioned for a thoracentesis. (From Elkin MK, Perry AG, Potter PA:* Nursing interventions and clinical skills, *St Louis, 1996, Mosby).*

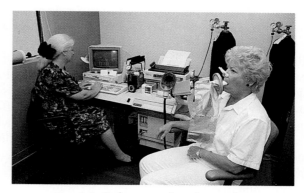

Fig. 4-2 *Pulmonary function testing.*

- *Pulmonary function tests*—Tests measure the amount of air moving in and out of the lungs (volume) and how much air the lungs can hold (capacity). The person takes as deep a breath as possible. Using a mouthpiece, the person blows into a machine (Fig. 4-2). The tests are used to evaluate persons at risk for lung diseases or postoperative pulmonary complications. They also are used to measure the progress of lung disease and its treatment. Fatigue is common after the tests. The person should rest after the procedure.

- *Arterial blood gases (ABGs)*—A radial or femoral artery is punctured to obtain arterial blood. Laboratory tests measure the amount of oxygen in the blood. Hemorrhage from the artery must be prevented. Pressure is applied to the artery for at least 5 minutes after the procedure. Pressure is applied longer if the person has blood clotting problems.

Pulse oximetry Pulse oximetry measures *(metry)* oxygen *(oxi)* concentration in arterial blood. **Oxygen concentration** is the amount (percent) of hemoglobin that contains oxygen. The normal range is 95% to 100%. For example, if 97% of all the hemoglobin (100%) carries O_2, tissues get enough oxygen. If only 90% of the hemoglobin contains O_2, tissues do not get enough oxygen to function. Measurements are used to prevent hypoxia and to evaluate treatment.

A sensor (or probe) is attached to the person's finger, toe, earlobe, nose, or forehead (Fig. 4-3). Two light beams on one side of the sensor pass through the tissues. A detector on the other side measures the amount of light passing through the tissues. The oximeter receives this information and measures the oxygen concentration. The value and the person's pulse rate are displayed on the monitor. Oximeters have alarms. The alarms sound if oxygen concentration is low, the pulse is too fast or slow, or other problems occur.

A

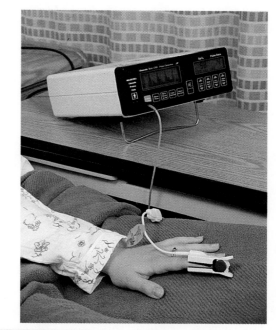

B

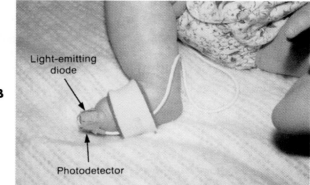

Light-emitting diode

Photodetector

Fig. 4-3 *A, A pulse oximetry sensor is attached to a person's finger. B, The sensor is attached to an infant's great toe. (B from Wong DL:* Whaley & Wong's nursing care of infants and children, *ed 5, St Louis, 1995, Mosby.)*

A good sensor site is needed. The RN tells you what site to use based on the person's condition. Swollen sites are avoided. So are sites with breaks in the skin. Finger and toe sites are avoided in persons with poor circulation.

Bright light, dark nail polish, and movements affect measurements. Place a towel over the sensor to block bright light. Remove nail polish or use another site. Movements from shivering, seizures, or tremors affect finger sensors. The earlobe is a better site for those with these problems. Blood pressure cuffs affect blood flow. If using a finger site, do not measure blood pressure on that side.

Report and record measurements accurately. Use the abbreviation SpO_2 when recording the oxygen concentration value (S = saturation, p = pulse, O_2 = oxygen).

Also report and record:

- The date and time
- What the person was doing at the time of the measurement
- Oxygen flow rate and the device used (p. 64)
- Reason for the measurement (routine or change in the person's condition)
- Other observations

Pulse oximetry does not lessen the need for good observations. The person's condition can change rapidly. You assist the RN in observing for signs and symptoms of hypoxia.

USING A PULSE OXIMETER

PRE-PROCEDURE

1 Review the procedure with the RN.
2 Ask the RN what site to use.
3 Explain the procedure to the person.
4 Collect the following:
- Oximeter and sensor
- Nail polish remover
- Cotton balls
- SpO_2 flow sheet
- Tape
- Towel
5 Identify the person. Check the ID bracelet with the assignment sheet. Provide for privacy.

PROCEDURE

6 Make sure the person is comfortable.
7 Remove nail polish using a cotton ball. (If a toe site is used, remove any nail polish).
8 Dry the site with a towel.
9 Clip or tape the sensor to the site. Make sure the site is dry.
10 Turn on the oximeter.
11 Check the person's pulse (apical or radial) with the pulse on the display. The pulses should be equal. Tell the RN if the pulses are not equal.
12 Read the SpO_2 on the display. Note the value on the flow sheet.
13 Leave the sensor in place for continuous monitoring. Otherwise, turn off the oximeter and remove the sensor.

POST-PROCEDURE

14 Make sure the person is comfortable.
15 Place the call bell within the person's reach.
16 Raise or lower bed rails as instructed by the RN.
17 Unscreen the person. Follow facility policy for soiled linen.
18 Return the pulse oximeter to its proper place if continuous monitoring is not ordered.
19 Wash your hands.
20 Report the SpO_2 and your other observations to the RN.

focus on children The sensor is attached to the sole of a foot, palm of the hand, finger, toe, or earlobe (see Fig. 4-3, *B*). If the child moves a lot, the earlobe is a better site.

focus on older persons Older persons often have poor circulation from aging or vascular disease. Blood flow to the toe or finger may be poor. Use the ear, nose, and forehead sites.

focus on home care Small hand-held oximetry units are available for home use. Instead of constant monitoring, oxygen concentration is often measured with vital signs. Because it is portable and used for many patients, you must make sure the pulse oximeter is accurate. After applying the sensor, check the person's pulse (radial or apical) with the displayed pulse. The pulse rates should be the same.

focus on children Breathing treatments and suctioning are often needed to produce a sputum specimen in infants and small children. The RN or respiratory therapist gives the breathing treatment. The RN suctions the trachea for the sputum specimen. The infant or child is likely to be uncooperative during suctioning. You can assist by holding the child's head and arms still.

focus on older persons Older persons may not have the strength to cough up sputum. Coughing is easier after postural drainage. Postural drainage involves draining secretions by gravity. Gravity causes fluids to flow down. Therefore the person is positioned so a lung part is lower than the airway (Fig. 4-4). Different positions are used depending on what part of the lungs are to be drained. The RN or respiratory therapist is responsible for postural drainage.

Collecting sputum specimens Respiratory disorders cause the lungs, bronchi, and trachea to secrete mucus. The mucus is called **sputum** when expectorated (expelled) through the mouth. Sputum is different from saliva. Saliva is a thin, clear liquid produced by the salivary glands in the mouth. Saliva is often called "spit."

Sputum specimens are studied for blood, microbes, and abnormal cells. The person coughs up sputum from the bronchi and trachea. This is often painful and difficult. Specimen collection is easier in the early morning when secretions are coughed up upon awakening. The person rinses the mouth with water. Rinsing decreases saliva and removes food particles. Mouthwash is not used before the procedure. It destroys some of the microbes in the mouth.

Collecting a sputum specimen can embarrass the person. Coughing and expectorating sounds can upset or nauseate other persons nearby. Also, sputum is unpleasant to look at. For these reasons, privacy is important. The specimen container is covered and placed in a bag. Some facilities use sputum containers that conceal the contents.

A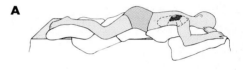

B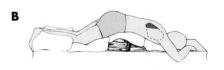

C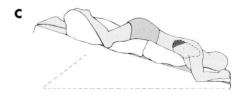

Fig. 4-4 *Some positions used for postural drainage. **A,** Draining the right upper lobe. **B,** Draining the right middle lobe. **C,** Draining the right lower lobe.* (From Potter PA, Perry AG: Fundamentals of nursing: concepts, process, and practice, ed 4. St Louis, 1997, Mosby.)

Collecting a Sputum Specimen

Pre-procedure

1 Explain the procedure to the person.
2 Wash your hands.
3 Collect the following:
   - Sputum specimen container
   - Tissues
   - Label
   - Laboratory requisition
   - Disposable bag
   - Disposable gloves

Procedure

4 Label the container.
5 Identify the person. Check the ID bracelet with the requisition slip.
6 Provide for privacy. If able, the person goes into the bathroom to obtain the specimen.
7 Ask the person to rinse the mouth out with clear water.
8 Put on the gloves.
9 Have the person hold the container. Only the outside of the container is touched.
10 Ask the person to cover the mouth and nose with tissues when coughing.
11 Ask him or her to take 2 or 3 deep breaths and cough up the sputum.
12 Have the person expectorate directly into the container (Fig. 4-5). Sputum should not touch the outside of the container.
13 Collect 1 to 2 tablespoons of sputum unless told to collect more.
14 Put the lid on the container immediately.
15 Place the container in the bag. Attach the requisition to the bag.
16 Remove the gloves.

Post-procedure

17 Make sure the person is comfortable and unscreened. Place the call bell within reach.
18 Wash your hands.
19 Take the bag to the laboratory.
20 Wash your hands.
21 Report the following to the RN:
   - The time the specimen was collected and taken to the laboratory
   - The amount of sputum collected
   - How easily the person raised the sputum
   - The consistency and appearance of sputum (see Box 4-2)
   - Any other observations

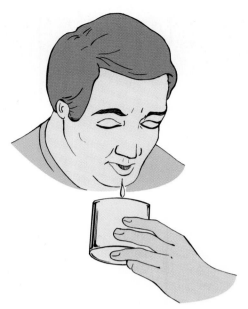

Fig. 4-5 *The person expectorates into the center of the specimen container.*

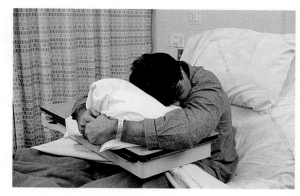

Fig. 4-6 *The person is in the orthopneic position. Note that a pillow is on the overbed table for the person's comfort.*

PROMOTING OXYGENATION

For the body to get enough oxygen, air must move deeply into the lungs. Air must reach the alveoli for the exchange of oxygen and carbon dioxide with the blood. Disease and injury can prevent air from reaching the alveoli. Secretions can congest lung tissue and the airway. Pain, immobility, and narcotics interfere with deep breathing and coughing up secretions. Therefore secretions collect in the respiratory system. They interfere with air movement and alveolar function in the affected part of the lung. Secretions also provide an environment for microbes. Infection is a threat.

The RN plans measures to meet the person's oxygen needs. The following measures are often included in nursing care plans.

Positioning

Breathing is usually easier in semi-Fowler's and Fowler's position. Persons with difficulty breathing often prefer to sit up in bed and lean forward over the overbed table. This is called the **orthopneic position.** *Ortho* means sitting or standing; *pnea* means breathing. You can increase the person's comfort by placing a pillow on the overbed table (Fig. 4-6).

Frequent position changes are important. Unless the doctor limits positioning, the person must not lie on one side for a long time. This prevents lung expansion on that side and allows secretions to pool. Position changes are usually done at least every 2 hours.

Coughing and Deep Breathing

Mucus is removed by coughing. Deep breathing promotes air movement into most parts of the lungs. Coughing and deep breathing exercises are helpful for persons with respiratory disorders. They are routinely done after surgery and are important for persons on bed rest. The exercises are painful after injury or surgery. The person may be afraid of breaking open an incision while coughing.

Coughing and deep breathing help prevent pneumonia and atelectasis. *Atelectasis* is the collapse of a portion of the lung. It occurs when mucus collects in the airway. Air cannot get to a part of the lung, and the lung collapses.

The frequency of coughing and deep breathing varies. Some doctors order the exercises every 1 or 2 hours while the person is awake. Others want them done 4 times a day. The RN tells you when coughing and deep breathing are done. You are told how many deep breaths and coughs the person should do.

ASSISTING THE PERSON WITH COUGHING AND DEEP BREATHING EXERCISES

PRE-PROCEDURE

1 Explain the procedure to the person.

2 Identify the person. Check the ID bracelet with the assignment sheet.

3 Provide for privacy.

PROCEDURE

4 Help the person to a comfortable sitting position: dangling, semi-Fowler's, or Fowler's.

5 Have the person deep breathe:

   a Have the person place the hands over the rib cage (Fig. 4-7).

   b Ask the person to exhale. Explain that when exhaling, the ribs should move as far down as possible.

   c Have the person take a deep breath. It should be as deep as possible. Remind the person to inhale through the nose.

   d Ask the person to hold the breath for 3 seconds.

   e Ask the person to exhale slowly through pursed lips (Fig. 4-8). The person should exhale until the ribs move as far down as possible.

   f Repeat this step 4 more times.

6 Ask the person to cough:

   a Have the person interlace the fingers over the incision (Fig. 4-9, *A*). The person can also hold a small pillow or folded towel over the incision (Fig. 4-9, *B*).

   b Have the person take in a deep breath as in step 5.

   c Ask the person to cough strongly twice with the mouth open.

POST-PROCEDURE

7 Assist the person to a comfortable position.

8 Raise or lower bed rails as instructed by the RN.

9 Place the call bell within reach.

10 Unscreen the person.

11 Report your observations to the RN:

   • The number of times the person coughed and deep breathed

   • How the person tolerated the procedure

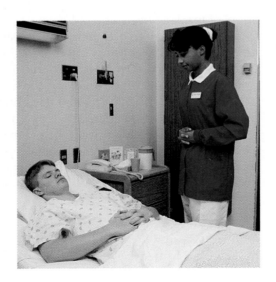

Fig. 4-7 *The hands are over the rib cage for deep breathing.*

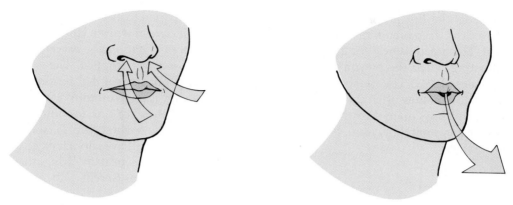

Fig. 4-8 *The person inhales through the nose and exhales through pursed lips during the deep breathing exercise.*

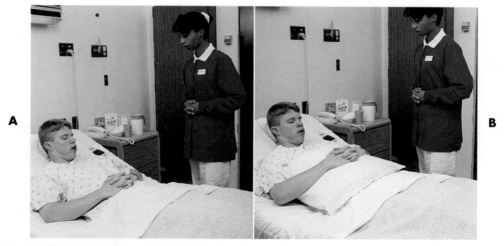

Fig. 4-9 *The person supports an incision for the coughing exercise. **A,** Fingers are interlaced over the incision. **B,** A small pillow is held over the incision.*

Incentive Spirometry

Incentive means to give encouragement. A *spirometer* is a machine that measures the amount (volume) of air inhaled. Thus incentive spirometry involves encouraging the person to inhale until reaching a preset volume of air. Balls or bars in the spirometer allow the person to see the movement of air when inhaling (Fig. 4-10).

The spirometer is placed upright. The person exhales normally and then seals the lips around a mouthpiece. The person takes in a slow, deep breath until the balls rise to the desired height. The breath is held for 2 to 6 seconds to keep the balls floating. Then the person removes the mouthpiece and exhales slowly. The person may cough at this time. The RN tells you how often the person needs incentive spirometry and how many breaths the person needs to take. Follow agency policy for cleaning and replacing disposable mouthpieces.

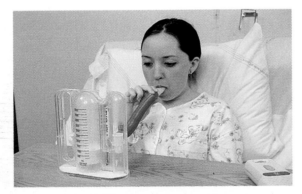

Fig. 4-10 *The person uses a spirometer.*

ASSISTING WITH OXYGEN THERAPY

Disease, injury, and surgery often interfere with breathing. The amount of oxygen in the blood may be less than normal (hypoxemia). If so, the doctor orders supplemental oxygen.

Oxygen is treated as a drug. The doctor orders the amount of oxygen to give and the device to use. The order also states if oxygen is given continuously or intermittently (periodically). *Continuous oxygen therapy* means that the oxygen is never stopped. That is, the administration of oxygen is not interrupted for any reason. *Intermittent oxygen therapy* is for symptom relief. Chest pain and exercise are common reasons for intermittent oxygen. The oxygen helps relieve chest pain. Persons with chronic respiratory diseases may have enough oxygen at rest. With mild exercise or activities of daily living, they become short of breath. Oxygen helps to relieve the shortness of breath.

You are not responsible for administering oxygen. The RN and respiratory therapist start and maintain oxygen therapy. You assist the RN in providing safe care to persons receiving oxygen.

Oxygen Sources

Oxygen is supplied through wall outlets, oxygen tanks, and oxygen concentrators. With the wall outlet (Fig. 4-11), O_2 is piped into each patient unit. Each unit is connected to a centrally located oxygen supply.

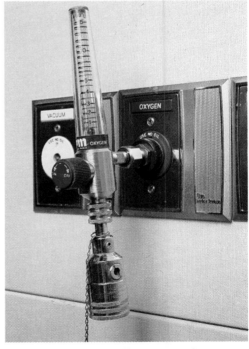

Fig. 4-11 *Wall oxygen outlet.*

The oxygen tank is portable. It is brought to the person's unit when the doctor orders oxygen therapy. Small tanks are used during emergencies and transfers. Some ambulatory persons need continuous oxygen. Portable tanks are used when walking (Fig. 4-12). The gauge on the tank tells how much oxygen is left in the tank (Fig. 4-13). Tell the RN if the tank is low.

Oxygen concentrators (Fig. 4-14) do not need an oxygen source (wall outlet or tank). The concentrator removes oxygen from the air. A power source is needed. If the concentrator is not portable, moving about is limited. The person stays close to the machine. A portable oxygen tank is needed in case of a power failure and for mobility.

focus on home care Oxygen tanks and oxygen concentrators are used in home care. The source ordered depends on the person's needs. The tank or concentrator is supplied by a medical supply company. Keep the company's name and phone number near the telephone.

The patient and family must practice safety measures where oxygen is used and stored. The safety measures to prevent fire are practiced (Box 4-3, p. 64). Also, the oxygen tank is kept away from open flames and heat sources. These include candles, gas stoves, heating ducts, radiators, heating pipes, space heaters, and kerosene heaters and lamps. Keep a fire extinguisher in the room. If a fire occurs, turn off the oxygen. Then get the person and other family members out of the home and call the fire department.

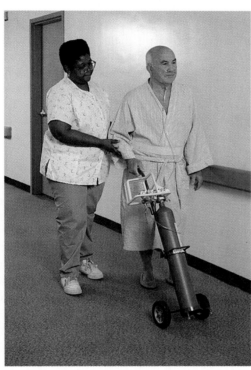

Fig. 4-12 *The person uses a portable oxygen tank during ambulation.*

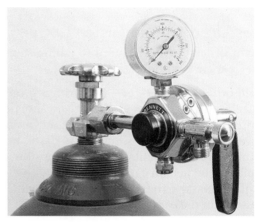

Fig. 4-13 *The gauge shows the amount of oxygen remaining in the tank.*

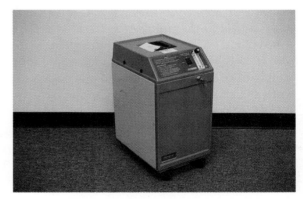

Fig. 4-14 *Oxygen concentrator.*

BOX 4-3 SAFETY RULES FOR FIRE AND USING OXYGEN

- Place "No Smoking" signs in the room and on the room door.
- Remove smoking materials from the room (cigarettes, cigars, pipes, matches, and lighters).
- Remove materials from the room that ignite easily (alcohol, nail polish remover, oils, greases).
- Keep oxygen tanks away from heat sources.

- Turn off electrical items before unplugging them.
- Use electrical equipment that is in good repair (razor, radio, TV, and others).
- Use only electrical equipment with three-prong plugs.
- Do not use materials that cause static electricity (wool and synthetic fabrics). ✳

Devices Used to Administer Oxygen

The doctor orders the device used to administer oxygen. These devices are common:

- *Nasal cannula* (Fig. 4-15)—two prongs project from the tubing. The prongs are inserted a short distance into the nostrils. The prongs point downward. This prevents drying of the sinuses. An elastic headband or tubing brought behind the ears keeps the cannula in place. The person can eat and talk with a cannula in place. Nasal irritation occurs with tight prongs. Pressure on the ears is possible.

- *Simple face mask* (Fig. 4-16)—covers the nose and mouth. The mask has small holes in the sides. Carbon dioxide escapes during exhalation. Room air enters during inhalation.

- *Partial-rebreathing face mask* (Fig. 4-17)—a reservoir bag is added to the simple face mask. The bag is for exhaled air. With inhalation, the person inhales oxygen and some of the exhaled air. Some room air also is inhaled. The bag should not totally deflate when the person inhales.

- *Nonrebreathing face mask* (Fig. 4-18)—prevents exhaled air from entering the reservoir bag. Exhaled air leaves through holes in the mask. When the person inhales, oxygen from the reservoir bag is inhaled. The bag must not totally collapse during exhalation.

- *Venturi mask* (Fig. 4-19)—allows precise amounts of oxygen to be given. Color-coded adapters indicate the amount of oxygen being delivered.

Special care is needed when masks are used. Masks make talking difficult. Listen carefully to what the person is saying. Moisture can build up under masks. Keep the person's face clean and dry to help prevent irritation from the mask. Masks are removed for eating. Usually oxygen is administered by nasal cannula during meals.

Oxygen Flow Rates

The amount of oxygen given is called the *flow rate*. This is ordered by the doctor. The flow rate is measured in liters per minute (L/min). The flow rate is anywhere from 2 to 15 liters of oxygen per minute. The flowmeter (see Fig. 4-11) is set for the desired rate. This is done by the RN or respiratory therapist.

The RN tells you what the flow rate is for the person. When giving care and checking patients, always check the flow rate. Tell the RN immediately if the flow rate is too high or too low. The flow rate is adjusted by an RN or respiratory therapist. Some states and facilities let assistive personnel adjust oxygen flow rates.

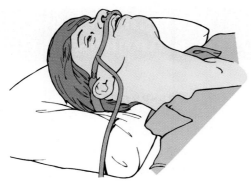

Fig. 4-15 *Nasal cannula.*

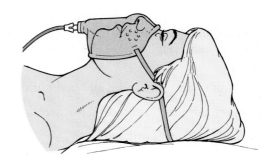

Fig. 4-16 *Simple face mask.*

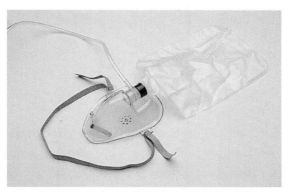

Fig. 4-17 *Partial-rebreathing face mask.*

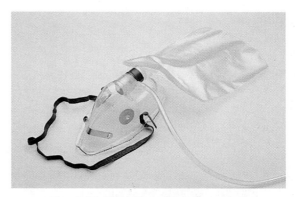

Fig. 4-18 *Nonrebreathing face mask.*

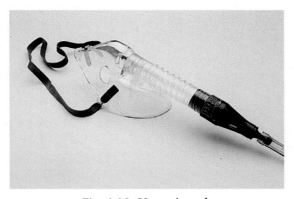

Fig. 4-19 *Venturi mask.*

Preparing for Oxygen Administration

Your job description may let you set up the oxygen administration system (Fig. 4-20). The RN tells you the following:

- The person's name and room and bed number
- The oxygen administration device ordered
- If humidification was ordered

Oxygen is a dry gas. If not humidified (made moist), oxygen dries the airway's mucous membranes. Distilled water is added to the humidifier to create water vapor. Oxygen tubing is attached to the humidifier. Oxygen picks up water vapor as it flows into the system. Bubbling in the humidifier means water vapor is being produced. If humidification is not ordered, distilled water and the humidifier are not used.

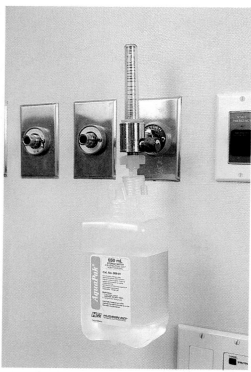

Fig. 4-20 *Oxygen administration system with humidifier.*

SETTING UP FOR OXYGEN ADMINISTRATION

PRE-PROCEDURE

1 Review the doctor's orders with the RN.

2 Wash your hands.

3 Collect the following:

- Oxygen administration device with connecting tubing
- Flowmeter
- Humidifier (if ordered)
- Distilled water (if using a humidifier)

PROCEDURE

4 Identify the person. Check the ID bracelet with the assignment sheet.

5 Explain to the person what you are going to do.

6 Make sure the flowmeter is in the *OFF* position.

7 Attach the flowmeter to the wall outlet.

8 Fill the humidifier with distilled water.

9 Attach the humidifier to the bottom of the flowmeter.

10 Attach the oxygen administration device and connecting tubing to the humidifier. *Do not set the flowmeter or apply the oxygen administration device on the person.*

POST-PROCEDURE

11 Discard packaging.

12 Make sure the cap is securely on the distilled water. Store it according to facility policy.

13 Make sure the person is comfortable and the call bell is within reach.

14 Tell the RN that you completed the procedure. *The RN will:*

- *Turn on the oxygen and set the flow rate*
- *Apply the oxygen administration device on the person*

15 Wash your hands.

Oxygen Safety

Remember, you assist the RN with oxygen therapy. You are not responsible for administering oxygen. You do not adjust the flow rate unless allowed by your state and facility. However, you must give safe care to persons receiving oxygen. Box 4-4 lists the rules for assisting with oxygen therapy. Also follow the rules in Box 4-3.

BOX 4-4 SAFETY RULES FOR OXYGEN THERAPY

- Never remove the device (cannula, mask) used to administer oxygen.
- Make sure the oxygen administration device is secure but not tight.
- Check for signs of irritation from the device. Check behind the ears, under the nose (cannula), and around the face (mask).
- Never shut off oxygen flow from the wall outlet, tank, or oxygen concentrator.
- Do not adjust the flow rate unless allowed by your state and facility.
- Notify the RN immediately if the flow rate is too high or too low.
- Make sure the humidifier is bubbling. Notify the RN immediately if the humidifier is not bubbling.
- Tape connecting tubing to the person's gown. Tubing must be secured in place.
- Make sure there are no kinks in the tubing.
- Make sure the person is not lying on any part of the tubing.
- Report signs and symptoms of hypoxia, respiratory distress, or abnormal breathing patterns to the RN immediately (see Boxes 4-1 and 4-2).
- Give oral hygiene as directed by the RN.
- Make sure the device is clean and free of mucus.
- Maintain an adequate water level in the humidifier. ✳

ARTIFICIAL AIRWAYS

Artificial airways keep the airway patent (open). They are used when:

- The airway is obstructed from disease, injury, secretions, or aspiration
- The person is semiconscious or unconscious
- The person is recovering from anesthesia
- The person needs mechanical ventilation (see p. 80)

Intubation is the process of inserting an artificial airway. Usually plastic, disposable airways are used. They come in adult, pediatric, and infant sizes. The following airways are common:

- *Oropharyngeal airway*—is inserted through the mouth and into the pharynx (Fig. 4-21, *A*, p. 68). An RN can insert the airway.
- *Nasopharyngeal airway*—is inserted through a nostril and into the pharynx (Fig. 4-21, *B*, p. 68). An RN can insert the airway.
- *Endotracheal tube*—is inserted through the mouth or nose and into the trachea (Fig. 4-21, *C*, p. 68). A doctor or RN with special training intubates using a lighted scope. A balloon (called a *cuff*) at the end of the tube is inflated to keep the airway in place.
- *Tracheostomy tube*—is inserted through a surgical incision (*ostomy*) into the trachea (*tracheal*) (Fig. 4-21, *D*, p. 68). Some tracheostomy tubes have cuffs. The cuff is inflated to keep the tube in place. The tracheostomy is done by a doctor.

You assist the RN in caring for persons with artificial airways. The person's vital signs are checked often. The person is observed for hypoxia and other respiratory signs and symptoms. If an airway comes out or is dislodged, tell the RN immediately. The person needs frequent oral hygiene. The RN tells you when and how to perform oral hygiene.

Talking is hard with oropharyngeal and nasopharyngeal airways. Persons with endotracheal tubes cannot speak. Some tracheostomy tubes allow the person to speak. Paper and pencils, magic slates, communication boards, and hand signals are ways to communiate.

Gagging and choking sensations are common with artificial airways. Imagine something in your mouth, nose, or throat. The person needs comforting and reassurance. Remind the person that the airway helps breathing. Use touch to show you care.

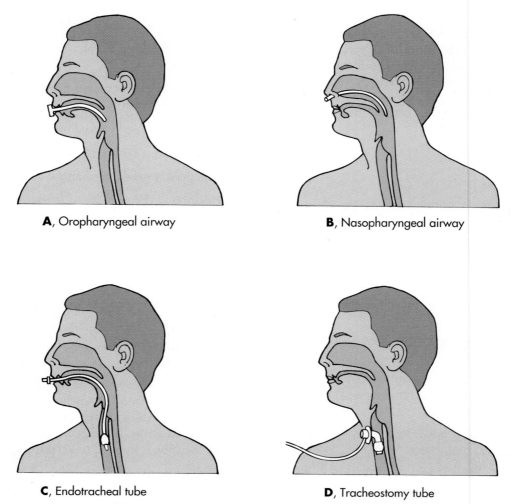

A, Oropharyngeal airway

B, Nasopharyngeal airway

C, Endotracheal tube

D, Tracheostomy tube

Fig. 4-21 *Artificial airways.* **A,** *Oropharyngeal airway.* **B,** *Nasopharyngeal airway.* **C,** *Endotracheal tube.* **D,** *Tracheostomy tube.*

Tracheostomies

Tracheostomies are temporary or permanent. They are temporary when the person requires mechanical ventilation (see p. 80). They are permanent when airway structures are surgically removed. Some cancers require removing airway structures. Sometimes a permanent tracheostomy is required when severe trauma injures the airway.

focus on children Some children are born with congenital defects. (*Congenitus* is a Latin word that means *to be born with.*) Therefore congenital defects are present at birth. Tracheostomies are needed for some congenital defects affecting the neck and airway. Some infections cause airway structures to swell. This obstructs airflow. Foreign body aspiration also obstructs airflow. These situations can require emergency tracheostomies.

Tracheostomy tubes are made of plastic or metal. A tracheostomy tube has three parts (Fig. 4-22): the outer tube, the inner tube, and obturator. *Cannula* is another word for tube. The inner and outer tubes are often called the *inner and outer cannulas.*

The obturator has a rounded end. It is used to insert the outer cannula. After the outer cannula is inserted, the obturator is removed. (The obturator is placed within easy reach in case the tracheostomy tube falls out and needs to be reinserted. It is taped to the wall or bedside stand.) The inner cannula is inserted and locked in place. The outer cannula is secured in place with ties around the person's neck or a Velcro collar. The inner cannula is removed for cleaning and mucus removal. This keeps the airway patent. The outer cannula is not removed.

Some plastic tracheostomy tubes do not have inner cannulas. These are used for persons who are suctioned often. With frequent suctioning, mucus does not stick to the cannula.

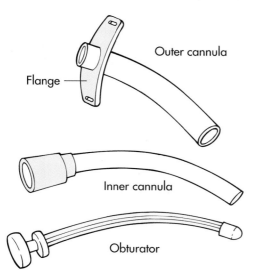

Fig. 4-22 *Parts of a tracheostomy tube.*

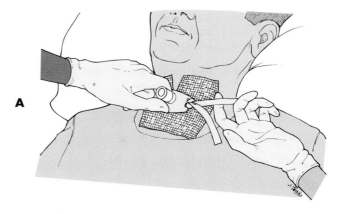

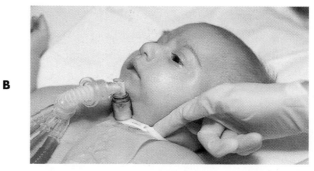

Fig. 4-23 *A, A finger is inserted under the ties. Note that a co-worker is holding the flange to prevent the tube from coming out. B, For children, only a fingertip is inserted under the ties. (B from Wong DL:* Whaley & Wong's nursing care of infants and children, *ed 5, St Louis, 1995, Mosby.)*

The cuffed tracheostomy tube provides a seal between the cannula and the trachea (see Fig. 4-21, *D*). This type is used with mechanical ventilation. The cuff prevents air from leaking around the tube. It also prevents aspiration. The RN or respiratory therapist inflates and deflates the cuff.

Securing tracheostomy tubes in place is important. The tube must not come out (extubation). If not secured properly, the tube could come out with coughing or if pulled on. Damage to the airway is possible if the tube is loose and moves up and down in the trachea.

The tracheostomy tube must remain patent (open). Some persons can cough secretions up and out of the tracheostomy. Others require suctioning (see p. 74).

Measures are needed to prevent aspiration. Nothing can enter the stoma. Otherwise the person can aspirate. The RN teaches the person and family the following:

- Make sure dressings do not have loose gauze or lint.
- Keep the stoma or tube covered when outside. Wear a stoma cover, scarf, or shirt or blouse that buttons at the neck. The cover prevents dust, insects, and other small particles from entering the stoma.
- Take tub baths instead of showers. If showers are taken, wear a shower guard and use a hand-held nozzle. Direct water away from the stoma.
- Be careful when shampooing. Ask another person to help you.
- Cover the stoma when shaving.
- Do not swim. Water will enter the tube or stoma.
- Wear a medical alert bracelet. Also carry a medical alert ID card.

Tracheostomy care Tracheostomy care involves cleaning the inner cannula, cleaning the stoma, and applying clean ties or Velcro collar. Cleaning the inner cannula removes mucus. This keeps the airway patent. A clean stoma and clean ties or collar help prevent infection at the tracheostomy site. Cleaning the stoma also helps prevent skin breakdown.

Some inner cannulas are disposable. They are used once and then discarded. The inner cannula is not cleaned. A new one is inserted.

The RN tells you when to do tracheostomy care. It may be done daily or every 8 to 12 hours. Tracheostomy care is done when there are excess secretions, the ties or collar are soiled, or the dressing is soiled or moist. A co-worker assists you. When the ties are removed, your co-worker holds the outer cannula in place. *If a co-worker is not available, do not remove the old ties or Velcro collar until you secure the new ones in place.* The ties or collar must be secure but not tight. A finger should slide under the ties or collar (Fig. 4-23).

Some states let assistive personnel give tracheostomy care when the stoma is permanent and healed. Before giving tracheostomy care, make sure that:

- Your state allows assistive personnel to perform the procedure

- The procedure is in your job description

- You have the necessary training

- You are familiar with the equipment

- You review the procedure with an RN

- An RN is available to answer questions and to supervise you

Call for the RN if the person shows signs and symptoms of hypoxia or respiratory distress during the procedure. Also call the RN if the outer cannula comes out during the procedure.

focus on children As with adults, the ties must be secure but not tight. Only a fingertip should slide under the ties (Fig. 4-23, *B*). Ties are too loose if you can slide your whole finger under them.

The tracheostomy care procedure is done with the help of a co-worker. The co-worker holds the child still. Your co-worker also positions the child's head so that the neck is slightly extended.

focus on home care A family member can help you during the procedure. Explain the procedure and what you want the family member to do.

Text continued on p. 74

GIVING TRACHEOSTOMY CARE

PRE-PROCEDURE

1 Review the procedure with the RN.
2 Ask a co-worker to help you. Explain what you want him or her to do.
3 Explain the procedure to the person.
4 Wash your hands.
5 Collect the following (some may be in a tracheostomy kit):
- Tracheostomy suction supplies (see p. 79)
- Sterile tracheostomy dressing
- 3 sterile 4 × 4 gauze square packages
- Hydrogen peroxide
- Sterile saline (to clean the inner cannula)
- 3 sterile cotton swab packages
- Sterile basin (to clean the inner cannula)
- Sterile brush (to clean the inner cannula)
- Tracheostomy ties or Velcro collar
- Disposable inner cannula (check with the RN)
- Scissors
- Sterile gloves (2 pair)
- Cotton twill tape
- Face shield
- Towel
6 Arrange supplies on the overbed table.
7 Identify the person. Check the ID bracelet with the assignment sheet. Provide for privacy.
8 Raise the bed to a level for good body mechanics. Make sure the far bed rail is up.
9 Position the patient supine or in Fowler's position.

GIVING TRACHEOSTOMY CARE—CONT'D

PROCEDURE

10 Suction the tracheostomy tube (see *Suctioning a Tracheostomy,* p. 79). Remember to wear a face shield.

11 Prepare a sterile field on the overbed table:

  a Open 2 sterile 4 × 4 gauze packages.

  b Open 2 sterile swab packages.

  c Pour sterile saline onto 1 sterile 4 × 4 gauze package and 1 sterile swab package.

  d Pour hydrogen peroxide onto 1 sterile 4 × 4 gauze package and 1 sterile swab package.

  e Open the sterile tracheostomy dressing package.

  f Open the sterile basin. Pour hydrogen peroxide into the basin. The peroxide should be about ³/₄ inch deep in the basin.

  g Open the sterile brush package.

12 Put on the sterile gloves.

13 Remove the inner cannula:

  a Unlock the inner cannula with your nondominant hand. Turn the lock counterclockwise. (This hand is now contaminated.)

  b Pull the inner cannula toward you with your non-dominant hand.

  c Drop the inner cannula into the basin with hydrogen peroxide. Or discard the cannula if it is disposable.

14 Clean the inner cannula. Go to step 15 if using a disposable inner cannula:

  a Clean the inside and outside of the cannula with the sterile brush (Fig. 4-24, p. 73). Use your dominant hand to clean with the brush.

  b Check the cannula to make sure all secretions and crusts are removed.

  c Pick up the bottle of sterile saline with your non-dominant hand.

  d Hold the cannula over the basin with hydrogen peroxide. (Use your dominant hand.)

  e Pour sterile saline over the inner cannula.

  f Tap the inner cannula against the inside of the sterile basin. This removes excess fluid to prevent aspiration.

15 Suction the outer cannula if secretions are present (see *Suctioning a Tracheostomy,* p. 79).

16 Replace the inner cannula with your dominant hand. Follow the direction of the tube's curve (Fig. 4-25, p. 73).

17 Lock the inner cannula in place. Turn the lock clockwise to an upright position.

18 Clean flange of the outer cannula with your dominant hand. Use sterile swabs and sterile 4 × 4 gauze moistened with hydrogen peroxide (Fig. 4-26). Use a new swab or gauze square for each stroke. *Make sure fluid does not enter the stoma.*

19 Remove the tracheostomy dressing with your non-dominant hand.

20 Clean under the stoma. Clean in circular motions away from the stoma (see Chapter 3). Use sterile swabs and sterile 4 × 4 gauze moistened with hydrogen peroxide. Use one swab or gauze square for each stroke. *Make sure fluid does not enter the stoma.*

21 Rinse the flange and under the stoma. Rinse outward from the stoma using sterile swabs and sterile 4 × 4 gauze moistened with sterile saline. *Make sure fluid does not enter the stoma.*

22 Pat dry the area around the stoma and the flange. Use the dry sterile swabs and the dry sterile 4 × 4 dressing.

23 Ask your co-worker to put on sterile gloves.

24 Have your co-worker hold the tracheostomy tube in place. The tube is held in place for steps 25–27.

25 Cut the ties or remove the Velcro collar following the manufacturer's instructions.

26 Change the ties or apply a new Velcro collar. Follow the manufacturer's instructions for applying the collar.

Continued

GIVING TRACHEOSTOMY CARE—CONT'D

PROCEDURE—CONT'D

Change the ties as follows:

a   Cut a length of twill tape about 24 to 30 inches long for the ties. Cut the tape longer if the person has a large neck.

b   Insert one end of the tie through the eyelet on the flange of the outer cannula (Fig. 4-27).

c   Slide the ends of the tie under the person's neck.

d   Bring the ends of the ties around to the eyelet on the other side of the flange.

e   Insert one tie through the eyelet.

f   Pull the ties so they are snug but not tight. You should be able to place a finger under the tie (see Fig. 4-23).

g   Tie the ties with two square knots at the side of the person's neck.

27   Apply the sterile tracheostomy dressing under the flange and clean ties (Fig. 4-28). Check the dressing for loose gauze and lint. Get a new dressing if necessary.

28   Ask your co-worker to let go of the outer cannula. Thank your co-worker for helping you.

29   Remove and discard the gloves and face shield.

POST-PROCEDURE

30   Make sure the person is comfortable.

31   Place the call bell within reach.

32   Lower the bed to its lowest horizontal position.

33   Raise or lower bed rails as instructed by the RN.

34   Unscreen the person.

35   Check to make sure that an extra tracheostomy tube is at the bedside. It must be the correct size for the person.

36   Empty the sterile basin.

37   Cap the hydrogen peroxide and saline bottles. Mark the date and time on each bottle. Store the bottles according to facility policy.

38   Discard used supplies and equipment according to facility policy.

39   Report your observations to the RN:

- The amount of secretions suctioned
- The color and consistency of secretions (see Box 4-2)
- The condition of the stoma and the skin around it
- How the person tolerated the procedure
- Any other observations

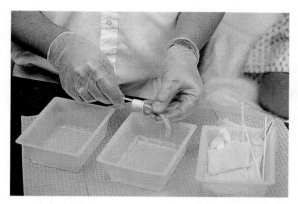

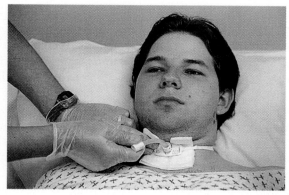

Fig. 4-24 *Clean the inner cannula with the brush. (From Elkin MK, Perry AG, Potter PA:* Nursing interventions and clinical skills, *St Louis, 1996, Mosby.)*

Fig. 4-25 *The inner cannula is replaced. (From Elkin MK, Perry AG, Potter PA:* Nursing interventions and clinical skills, *St Louis, 1996, Mosby.)*

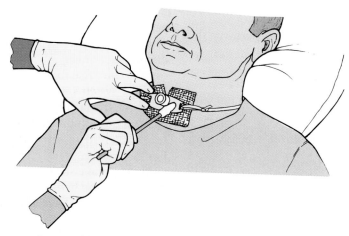

Fig. 4-26 *The outer flange of the tracheostomy tube is cleaned. A coworker holds the tracheostomy tube in place as in Step 24.*

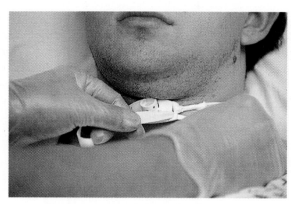

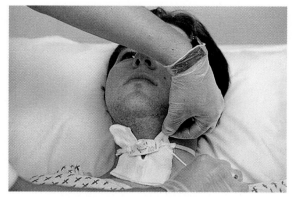

Fig. 4-27 *The tie is inserted through an eyelet on the flange. Note that the old ties are still in place when performing the procedure by yourself. (From Elkin MK, Perry AG, Potter PA:* Nursing interventions and clinical skills, *St Louis, 1996, Mosby.)*

Fig. 4-28 *The tracheostomy dressing is applied under the flange and clean ties. (From Elkin MK, Perry AG, Potter PA:* Nursing interventions and clinical skills, *St Louis, 1996, Mosby.)*

SUCTIONING THE AIRWAY

Injury and illness often cause secretions to collect in the upper airway. Removing the secretions is necessary so air can flow into and out of the airway. Retained secretions obstruct the airway. They provide an environment for microbes and interfere with oxygen and carbon dioxide exchange. Hypoxia occurs if secretions are not removed. Usually coughing removes the secretions. Sometimes the person cannot cough or the cough is too weak to remove secretions. Then suctioning is necessary.

Suction is the process of withdrawing or sucking up fluid (secretions). A tube is connected to a suction source (wall outlet or suction machine) at one end and to a suction catheter at the other end. The catheter is inserted into the airway. Secretions are withdrawn through the catheter.

States and facilities vary about the role of assistive personnel in airway suctioning. Before you perform suctioning procedures, make sure that:

- Your state allows assistive personnel to perform the procedure

- The task is in your job description

- You know how to use the facility's equipment and supplies

- You review the procedure with the RN before you begin

- An RN is available to answer your questions and to supervise you

Suctioning Routes

The nose, mouth, and pharynx make up the upper airway. The trachea and bronchi are the lower parts of the airway.

The *oropharyngeal* route involves suctioning the mouth *(oro)* and pharynx *(pharyngeal)*. The suction catheter is passed through the mouth and into the pharynx. The *nasopharyngeal* route involves suctioning the nose *(naso)* and pharynx *(pharyngeal)*. The suction catheter is passed through the nose and into the pharynx. These routes are used for persons who cannot expectorate or swallow secretions after coughing. Some states let assistive personnel do oral pharyngeal suctioning.

Lower airway suctioning is done through an endotracheal tube or a tracheostomy tube (see p. 67). Some states allow assistive personnel to suction permanent tracheostomies.

Safety Measures

If not done correctly, suctioning can seriously harm the person. Suctioning removes oxygen from the airway. Therefore the person does not get a fresh supply of oxygen during suctioning. Hypoxia and life-threatening complications can arise from the respiratory, cardiovascular, and nervous systems. Cardiac arrest can occur. Infection and injury to the airway's mucous membranes also are possible. You need to understand the principles and safety measures involved in safe suctioning. These are described in Box 4-5.

Always make sure needed suction equipment and supplies are at the bedside. When the person needs suctioning you do not have time to collect supplies from the supply area.

focus on children Suctioning procedures may frighten children. They need clear explanations about the procedure. As with other procedures, you may need someone to control the child's head and arm movements. A co-worker or family member can hold the child still.

focus on home care Agency policies differ about cleaning or changing the suction container. Some change the container every 24 hours. Others require daily cleaning of the container with hot water and soap. Follow agency policies for discarding or cleaning suction catheters, connecting tubing, and containers.

BOX 4-5 PRINCIPLES AND SAFETY MEASURES FOR SUCTIONING

- Do not suction a person unless the RN tells you to do so. Even if oropharyngeal suctioning or tracheostomy suctioning is included in your job description, the person's condition may require the care of an RN.
- Review the procedure with the RN. Make sure the RN is available if you have questions or have problems.
- Suctioning is done as needed *(prn)*. Coughing and signs and symptoms of respiratory distress signal the need for suctioning. The RN tells you what signs to look for in each person. Suctioning is not done at scheduled intervals.
- Standard Precautions and the Bloodborne Pathogen Standard are followed. Remember, secretions can contain blood and are potentially infectious.
- The mouth is clean, not sterile. Microbes enter the mouth through breathing, eating and drinking. Sterile technique is not required for oropharyngeal suctioning.
- Sterile technique is used when suctioning a tracheostomy (see Chapter 2).
- Use the catheter size as directed by the RN. Airway injury can occur if the catheter is too large.
- Limit the amount of suction as directed by the RN. Wall suction pressures usually are limited to 80 to

120 mm Hg in adults (80 to 100 mm Hg in children). Injury and complications are possible when suction pressure is too great.
- Do not apply suction while inserting the catheter. When suction is applied, air is sucked out of the person's airway.
- Clear the catheter with water or saline after removal.
- Insert the catheter smoothly. This helps prevent injury to the mucous membranes.
- Pass (insert) a suction catheter no more than 3 times. The risk of injury increases each time the suction catheter is passed.
- Check the person's pulse, respirations, and pulse oximeter before, during, and after the procedure. Also observe the person's level of consciousness. Call for the RN immediately if any of the following occur:
  * A drop in pulse rate or a pulse rate less than 60 beats per minute
  * Irregular cardiac rhythms
  * A drop or rise in blood pressure
  * Respiratory distress
  * A drop in the SpO_2 (see p. 56) ☀

Oropharyngeal Suctioning

Take no more than 10 to 15 seconds to complete a suction cycle. One complete cycle involves inserting the catheter, suctioning, and removing the catheter. (Hold your breath during the suction cycle. This helps you experience what the person feels during suctioning.)

Some patients have large amounts of thick secretions. The Yankauer suction catheter is often used for these persons (Fig. 4-29). It is larger and stiffer than other suction catheters.

Text continued on p. 78

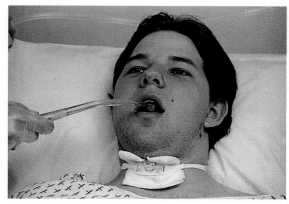

Fig. 4-29 *The Yankauer suction catheter. (From Elkin MK, Perry AG, Potter PA:* Nursing interventions and clinical skills, *St Louis, 1996, Mosby.)*

OROPHARYNGEAL SUCTIONING

PRE-PROCEDURE

1 Review the procedure with the RN.

2 Wash your hands.

3 Collect the following:

- Suction catheter (the RN tells you the kind and size)
- Connecting tubing
- Water (about 100 ml)
- Clean basin
- Suction machine (if no wall outlet suction)
- Disposable gloves
- Face shield if the person is likely to cough
- Towel

4 Identify the person. Check the ID bracelet with the assignment sheet.

5 Explain the procedure to the person.

6 Provide for privacy.

7 Raise the bed for good body mechanics. Make sure the far bed rail is raised.

PROCEDURE

8 Position the person in semi-Fowler's position. Turn his or her head toward you.

9 Place the towel under the person's chin and across the chest.

10 Wash your hands. Make sure both bed rails are raised before leaving the bedside. Lower the rail near you when you return to the person.

11 Put on the gloves. Also put on the face shield if needed.

12 Fill the basin with water.

13 Turn on the suction. The RN tells you what suction pressure to use.

14 Attach the connecting tubing to the wall suction or suction machine.

15 Attach the suction catheter to the connecting tubing (Fig. 4-30).

16 Check equipment function. Suction some water out of the basin.

17 Remove the oxygen mask if the person is using one.

18 Insert the suction catheter into the person's mouth along the gum line to the pharynx (Fig. 4-31).

19 Apply suction as you move the catheter along the gum lines and around the mouth.

20 Remove the catheter.

21 Rinse the catheter and connecting tubing. Rinse by suctioning a small amount of water from the basin.

22 Repeat steps 18 through 21 no more than two times.

23 Reapply the oxygen mask.

24 Clear the catheter and connecting tubing of secretions. Suction water from the basin until the tubing is clear.

25 Turn off the suction.

26 Disconnect the catheter from the connecting tubing.

27 Follow facility policy for reusing or discarding the catheter and suction container.

28 Remove the towel.

29 Remove and discard your gloves.

OROPHARYNGEAL SUCTIONING—CONT'D

POST-PROCEDURE

30 Make sure the person is comfortable. Place the call bell within the person's reach.

31 Lower the bed to its lowest horizontal position. Raise or lower bed rails as instructed by the RN.

32 Unscreen the person.

33 Empty the basin. Follow facility policy for reusing or discarding the basin.

34 Discard used supplies.

35 Wash your hands.

36 Report your observations to the RN:
- The amount of secretions suctioned
- The color and consistency of secretions (see Box 4-2)
- Signs and symptoms of hypoxia or respiratory distress
- How the person tolerated the procedure
- Any other observations

37 Collect supplies used during the procedure. Replace them at the bedside.

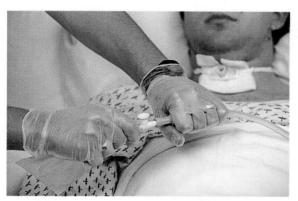

Fig. 4-30 *The suction catheter is attached to the connecting tubing. (From Elkin MK, Perry AG, Potter PA:* Nursing interventions and clinical skills, *St Louis, 1996, Mosby.)*

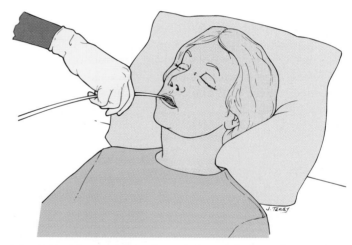

Fig. 4-31 *The suction catheter is inserted along the gum line.*

Tracheostomy Suctioning

When the person is seriously ill or requires mechanical ventilation (see p. 80), you can assist the RN with suctioning the tracheostomy. The RN may ask you to perform the procedure when:

- The person's condition is stable and not likely to change suddenly

- The tracheostomy is healed

Hypoxia is a risk during suctioning. Remember, the person does not receive oxygen when the suction catheter is inserted. Also, suction removes air out of the airway. Therefore the person's lungs are hyperventilated before applying suction. To *hyperventilate* means to give extra *(hyper)* breaths *(ventilate)*. This is done with a manual resuscitation or Ambu bag (Fig. 4-32). The Ambu bag is attached to an oxygen source. The oxygen delivery device is removed from the tracheostomy tube. The Ambu bag is attached to the tracheostomy tube. The bag is compressed (squeezed) as the person inhales. Three to five breaths are given as directed by the RN.

Both hands are used to compress the Ambu bag. You wear sterile gloves to hold and use the suction catheter. Therefore you cannot touch the Ambu bag. A co-worker is needed to help you. The co-worker uses the Ambu bag during the procedure.

Remember, an oxygen source is attached to the Ambu bag. Oxygen is treated like a drug. Assistive personnel are not allowed to administer drugs. Therefore you need to check if your state and facility allow you to use an Ambu bag attached to an oxygen source. It may be necessary for an RN or respiratory therapist to hyperventilate the lungs during the suction procedure. Remember, it takes two staff members to suction a tracheostomy. By having an RN hyperventilate the lungs, you are doing what your state and job description allow (suctioning). Because the RN administers the oxygen, you are not functioning beyond the limits of your role. The RN is with you if problems arise but able to do other things while you tend to pre-procedure and post-procedure activities.

Ask the RN about the length of time to apply suction. Some facilities limit suctioning to 10 seconds. Others allow 10 to 15 seconds for the suction cycle (inserting the catheter, applying suction, and removing the catheter). Make sure you clearly understand the RN's directions. You must know the difference between the length of time for applying suction and the length of time for the suction cycle.

focus on children For infants and children, suction is applied no longer than 5 seconds.

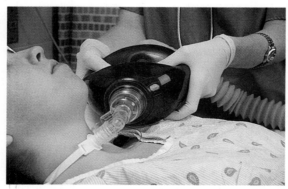

Fig. 4-32 *The Ambu bag. Two hands are used to compress the bag.*

SUCTIONING A TRACHEOSTOMY

PRE-PROCEDURE

1 Review the procedure with the RN.

2 Ask an RN or respiratory therapist to perform the hyperventilation function.

3 Wash your hands.

4 Collect the following:

- Sterile suction catheter (the RN tells you the kind and size)
- Connecting tubing
- Sterile water or sterile saline (about 100 ml)
- Sterile basin
- Suction machine (if no wall outlet suction)
- Sterile gloves
- Face shield
- Sterile drape
- Ambu bag
- Leakproof bag

5 Identify the person. Check the ID bracelet with the assignment sheet.

6 Explain the procedure to the person.

7 Provide for privacy.

8 Arrange equipment on the bedside table.

9 Raise the bed for good body mechanics. Make sure the far bed rail is raised.

PROCEDURE

10 Position the person in semi-Fowler's position. Turn his or her head toward you.

11 Wash your hands. Make sure both bed rails are raised before leaving the bedside. Lower the bed rail near you when you return to the person.

12 Open the sterile towel. Place it across the person's chest.

13 Open the sterile basin.

14 Pour the sterile water or saline into the basin.

15 Turn on the suction. The RN tells you what suction pressure to use.

16 Attach the connecting tubing to the wall suction or suction machine.

17 Open the sterile suction catheter package. Do not let the suction catheter touch any nonsterile surface.

18 Attach the suction catheter to the connecting tubing. Touch only the connecting end of the catheter.

19 Put on the face shield.

20 Put on the sterile gloves.

21 Pick up the suction catheter with your dominant hand. Hold the catheter with your thumb and forefinger.

22 Check equipment function. Suction some water or saline out of the basin.

23 Ask the RN or respiratory therapist to hyperventilate the person's lungs.

24 Insert the suction catheter into the tracheostomy. Insert the catheter until the person coughs or you feel resistance (usually about 6 inches for adults). *Do not apply suction.*

25 Pull the catheter back about $\frac{1}{2}$ inch (1 to 2 cm). *Do not apply suction.*

26 Apply suction intermittently for no more than 10 seconds (5 seconds in children). Intermittent suction means that you alternate covering and uncovering the thumb port (Fig. 4-33, p. 80). Use your nondominant hand to cover and uncover the thumb port.

27 Rotate the catheter, and slowly withdraw it as you apply intermittent suction. Rotate the catheter by rolling it between your thumb and forefinger (see Fig. 4-33).

28 Remove the catheter after 10 seconds. Release the suction by uncovering the thumb port.

29 Ask the RN or respiratory therapist to hyperventilate the person's lungs.

30 Rinse the catheter and connecting tubing. Rinse by suctioning a small amount of water from the basin.

31 Wait 1 to 3 minutes before repeating steps 23 through 30. Repeat the steps no more than 2 times.

32 Ask the RN or respiratory therapist to connect the oxygen delivery device to the tracheostomy.

Continued

SUCTIONING A TRACHEOSTOMY—CONT'D

PROCEDURE—CONT'D

33 Clear the catheter and connecting tubing of secretions. Suction water or saline from the basin until the tubing is clear.

34 Disconnect the catheter from the connecting tubing.

35 Roll the catheter into a ball in your hand or wrap it around your gloved hand.

36 Remove the sterile glove on the hand holding the catheter. The catheter is inside the glove as the glove is pulled off.

37 Put the glove with the catheter in your other hand.

38 Pull the glove over the glove in your hand.

39 Discard the gloves and catheter into a leakproof bag.

40 Turn off the suction.

41 Remove the sterile towel. Discard it into the leakproof bag.

POST-PROCEDURE

42 Make sure the person is comfortable. Place the call bell within the person's reach.

43 Lower the bed to its lowest horizontal position. Raise or lower bed rails as instructed by the RN.

44 Unscreen the person.

45 Disconnect the Ambu bag from the oxygen source.

46 Empty the basin. Follow facility policy for reprocessing or discarding the basin.

47 Remove and discard the face shield.

48 Wash your hands.

49 Report your observations to the RN:
- The amount of secretions suctioned
- The color and consistency of secretions (see Box 4-2)
- Signs and symptoms of hypoxia or respiratory distress
- How the person tolerated the procedure
- Any other observations

50 Collect supplies used during the procedure. Replace them at the bedside. Make sure a sterile tracheostomy tube is at the bedside. It must be the correct size for the person.

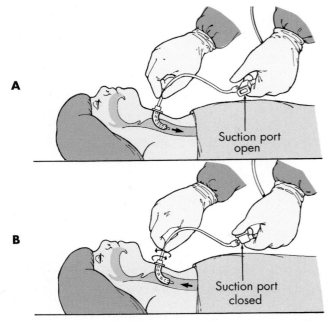

A

Suction port open

B

Suction port closed

*Fig. 4-33 Intermittent suction is applied. **A,** The thumb port is uncovered. **B,** The thumb port is covered. (From Wong DL: Whaley & Wong's nursing care of infants and children, ed 5, St Louis, 1995, Mosby.)*

MECHANICAL VENTILATION

Weak muscle effort, airway obstruction, and damaged lung tissue cause hypoxia. Central nervous system diseases and injuries can affect the respiratory center in the brain. Nerve damage can interfere with messages being sent between the lungs and the brain. Drug overdose can depress the brain. These and other respiratory problems are so severe that some patients cannot breathe on their own. Or they cannot maintain enough oxygen in the blood. These persons often need mechanical ventilation. *Mechanical ventilation* is using a machine to move air into and out of the lungs (Fig. 4-34). Oxygen enters the lungs, and carbon dioxide leaves the lungs.

Persons on mechanical ventilation have artificial airways. Depending on the person's problems, an endotracheal tube or tracheostomy tube is used. You assist the RN with the person's care.

Ventilators have alarms that warn when something is wrong. One alarm is for when the person gets discon-

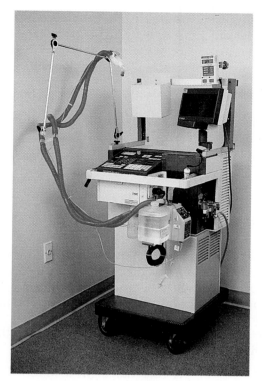

Fig. 4-34 *A mechanical ventilator.*

nected from the ventilator. *When any alarm sounds, first check to see if the person's endotracheal tube or tracheostomy tube is attached to the ventilator. If it is disconnected, attach the tube to the ventilator.* Then notify the RN immediately about the alarm. Do not reset alarms. Remember, the person is on a ventilator because of respiratory difficulties. The person can die if not connected to the ventilator.

Persons needing mechanical ventilation are seriously ill. They often have other problems and injuries. Their reactions to mechanical ventilation are many. Some are confused, disoriented, or unable to think clearly. Many are frightened by the machine and fear dying. Some feel relief when their bodies get enough oxygen. Many fear having to remain on the machine for life. Mechanical ventilation can be painful for those with chest injuries or chest surgery. Tubes and hoses restrict movement, adding to the person's discomfort.

The RN may ask you to assist with the person's care. The following are important aspects of the person's care:

- Keep the call bell within the person's reach.

- Make sure there is enough slack on hoses and connecting tubing. They should not pull on the endotracheal or tracheostomy tube.

- Answer call bells promptly. Remember, the person depends on others for basic needs.

- Explain who you are and what you are going to do whenever you enter the room.

- Orient the person to day, date, and time.

- Tell the RN immediately if the person shows signs of respiratory distress or discomfort.

- Do not change any settings on the ventilator or reset alarms.

- Provide a means of communication. Remember, the person on mechanical ventilation cannot talk.

- Use established hand or eye signals for "yes" and "no." All health team members (nursing staff, doctors, respiratory therapists, and others) and the family must use the same signals. Otherwise, communication does not occur.

- Ask questions that have simple answers. The person may not have the strength to write out long responses.

- Be careful what you say when within the person's hearing distance. The person may pay close attention to what is being said. Do not say anything that could upset the person.

- Watch your nonverbal communication. Although seriously ill and unable to speak, the person may be very aware of nonverbal messages. Avoid communicating worry and concern to the person.

- Take time to comfort and reassure the person. Tell the person what you are going to do and why. Also tell the person about such things as the weather, pleasant news events, and gifts and cards.

- Meet the person's basic needs for personal and oral hygiene, elimination, and activity (repositioning, range-of-motion exercises, sitting in a chair) as directed by the RN.

- Apply a moist wash cloth or lubricant to the person's lips as directed by the RN. This helps prevent the lips from drying and cracking.

- Use touch to reassure and comfort the person.

- Tell the person when you are leaving the room and when you will be back.

focus on long-term care Often patients are taken off the ventilator within hours or days of needing the device. However, some persons need the ventilator for longer periods. These patients may require long-term or subacute care. Often the person needs to be weaned from the ventilator. That is, the person needs to breathe without the ventilator. It may take several weeks to get the person off the ventilator. The respiratory therapist and RN plan the weaning process.

Home care is often arranged for ventilator-dependent persons. The RN teaches you how to care for each patient. You may be asked to give tracheostomy care and to suction the person. Family members also are taught how to assist with the person's care. Always make sure that an RN is available by phone when you are in the person's home. Make sure delegated tasks are allowed by your state and agency.

CHEST TUBES

When the chest is entered, air, blood, or fluid can collect in the pleural space (sac or cavity). Chest entry occurs with chest surgery or injury. **Pneumothorax** is the collection of air *(pneumo)* in the pleural space *(thorax)*. **Hemothorax** is the collection of blood *(hemo)* in the pleural space *(thorax)*. **Pleural effusion** is the collection of fluid *(effusion)* in the plueral space.

Pressure caused by the collection of air, blood, or fluid collapses the lung. Air cannot reach the affected aveoli. O_2 and CO_2 are not exchanged at the alveoli. Respiratory distress and hypoxia result. Sometimes there is pressure on the heart. This affects the heart's ability to pump blood and is a life-threatening problem.

The doctor inserts chest tubes to remove the air, fluid, or blood (Fig. 4-35). The sterile procedure is done in surgery, in the emergency room, or at the bedside. An RN assists with the procedure.

The chest tubes are attached to a drainage system (Fig. 4-36). The system must be airtight so that air does not enter the pleural space. Water-seal drainage is used to keep the system airtight (Fig. 4-37). This is done as follows:

- A chest tube is attached to connecting tubing.

- Connecting tubing is then attached to a tube in the drainage container.

- The tube in the drainage container extends under water. The water prevents air from entering the chest tube and then the pleural space.

A one-, two-, or three-bottle system or a disposable system is used (see Fig. 4-37). Disposable systems are common. Bottles are shown in Figure 4-37 to give you a clearer understanding of how the system works. Sometimes suction is applied to the drainage system.

When caring for persons with chest tubes, you need to:

- Keep the drainage system below the level of the person's chest.

- Measure the person's vital signs as directed by the RN. Report any changes in vital signs immediately.

- Report signs and symptoms of hypoxia and respiratory distress to the RN immediately; also report patient complaints of pain or difficulty breathing.

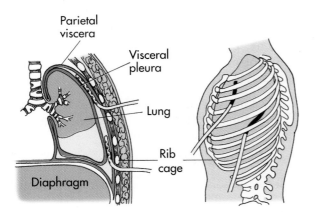

Fig. 4-35 *Chest tubes inserted into the pleural space. (From Elkin MK, Perry AG, Potter PA: Nursing interventions and clinical skills, St Louis, 1996, Mosby.)*

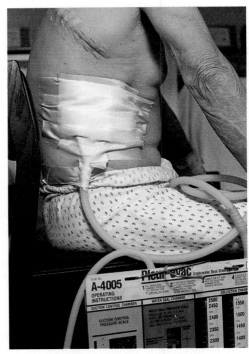

Fig. 4-36 *Chest tubes attached to a disposable water-seal drainage system. (From Elkin MK, Perry AG, Potter PA: Nursing interventions and clinical skills, St Louis, 1996, Mosby.)*

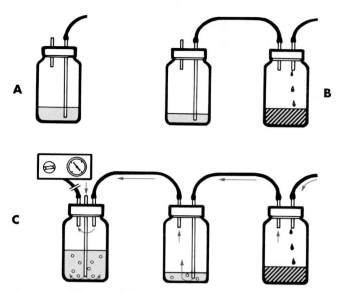

Fig. 4-37 *Water-seal drainage systems.* **A,** *One-bottle system.* **B,** *Two-bottle system.* **C,** *Three-bottle system with suction.* (*From Potter PA, Perry AG:* Fundamentals of nursing: concepts, process, and practice, *ed 4, St. Louis, 1997, Mosby.*)

- Keep connecting tubing coiled on the bed. Allow enough slack so the chest tubes are not dislodged when the person moves. If tubing hangs in loops, drainage collects in the loop.

- Make sure the tubing is not kinked. Kinking obstructs the chest tube causing air, blood, or fluid to collect in pleural space.

- Observe chest drainage. Immediately report to the RN any change in chest drainage. This includes increases in drainage or the appearance of bright red drainage.

- Record chest drainage according to facility policy.

- Turn and position the person as directed by the RN. The person must be turned carefully and gently to prevent the chest tubes from dislodging.

- Assist the person with coughing and deep breathing as directed by the RN. Also assist with incentive spirometry as directed.

- Note bubbling activity in the drainage system. Tell the RN immediately if the bubbling increases, decreases, or stops.

- Tell the RN immediately if any part of the system is loose or disconnected.

- Make sure petrolatum gauze is at the bedside in case a chest tube comes out.

- Call for help immediately if a chest tube comes out. Cover the insertion site with sterile petrolatum gauze. Stay with the person until an RN arrives. Follow the RN's directions.

CARDIOPULMONARY RESUSCITATION

Persons with respiratory injuries and problems are at risk for respiratory and cardiac arrest. Facility policy will require you to be certified in basic life support procedures. Such procedures include cardiopulmonary resuscitation (CPR). The American Heart Association, National Safety Council, and the American Red Cross have courses in basic life support. Your training program may include one of these courses. They also are available through many community agencies.

SUMMARY

You assist nurses in helping patients meet their oxygen needs. Oxygen is necessary for survival. Without it, a person dies. With inadequate oxygen, organ damage occurs. Serious illnesses and disabilities result.

Patients may need oxygen therapy, artificial airways, mechanical ventilators, or chest tubes. The RN plans nursing care to meet the person's basic needs. You are likely to assist with the person's care. You need to follow the person's nursing care plan, practice safety measures, and make accurate observations. Promptly report your observations to the RN. The person's condition can change rapidly.

Collecting sputum specimens and assisting with coughing and deep breathing exercises are common tasks for assistive personnel. Some states and facilities allow assistive personnel to assist with pulse oximetry, tracheostomy care, and suctioning. Tracheostomy care and suctioning are complex tasks. Serious harm to the person can result if the procedures are not performed properly. Inaccurate pulse oximetry measurements also are harmful. Before performing these procedures, make sure your state allows you to perform them. They must be in your job description, and you need to have training and supervision. Always make sure that an RN is available to answer your questions and to supervise you.

REVIEW QUESTIONS

Circle the best *answer.*

1 Alcohol and narcotics affect oxygen needs because they
   a Depress the brain
   b Are pollutants
   c Cause allergies
   d Cause a pneumothorax

2 Hypoxia is
   a A deficiency of oxygen in the blood
   b The amount of hemoglobin that contains oxygen
   c A deficiency of oxygen in the cells
   d The lack of oxygen

3 One of the earliest signs of hypoxia is
   a Cyanosis
   b Increased pulse and respiratory rates
   c Restlessness
   d Dyspnea

4 A person can breathe deeply and comfortably only while sitting or standing. This is called
   a Biot's respirations
   b Orthopnea
   c Bradypnea
   d Kussmaul's respirations

5 The person will probably need to rest after
   a A chest x-ray
   b A lung scan
   c Arterial blood gases
   d Pulmonary function tests

6 A person has pulse oximetry. The person's SpO$_2$ is 98%. Which is *true*?
   a The machine is not accurate.
   b The person's pulse is 98 beats per minute.
   c The measurement is within normal range.
   d The person needs suctioning.

7 Which is not a site for a pulse oximetry sensor?
   a Toe
   b Finger
   c Ear lobe
   d Upper arm

8 The best time to collect a sputum specimen is
   a On awakening
   b After meals
   c At bedtime
   d After suctioning

9 Before collecting a sputum specimen, you should
   a Ask the person to use mouthwash
   b Ask the person to rinse the mouth with clear water
   c Ask the person to brush the teeth
   d Apply lubricant to the person's lips

10 You are assisting a person with coughing and deep breathing. Which is *false*?
   a The person inhales through pursed lips.
   b The person needs to be in a comfortable sitting position.
   c The person inhales deeply through the nose.
   d The person holds a small pillow over an incision.

11 Which is useful for deep breathing?
   a Pulse oximeter
   b Incentive spirometry
   c Chest tubes
   d Partial-rebreathing mask

12 You are assisting with oxygen therapy. You can
   a Turn the oxygen on and off
   b Start the oxygen
   c Decide what device to use
   d Make sure the connecting tubing is secure and free of kinks

13 A person has a tracheostomy. Which is *false*?
   a A nondisposable inner cannula is removed for cleaning.
   b The obturator is inserted after the outer cannula.
   c The outer cannula must be secured in place.
   d The person must be protected from aspiration.

14 A person has a tracheostomy. The person can do the following *except*
   a Shampoo
   b Shave
   c Shower with a hand-held nozzle
   d Swim

REVIEW QUESTIONS—CONT'D

15 You are giving tracheostomy care by yourself. The old ties are removed after
   a Removing the inner cannula
   b Cleaning the flange and stoma
   c Removing the dressing
   d Securing the new ties

16 These statements are about oropharyngeal suctioning. Which is *true?*
   a Suction is applied while inserting the catheter.
   b Suctioning is done every two hours.
   c A suction cycle is no more than 10 to 15 seconds.
   d The mouth is considered sterile.

17 Oropharyngeal suctioning requires
   a Following Standard Precautions and the Bloodborne Pathogen Standard
   b Sterile technique
   c An artificial airway
   d All of the above

18 A child has a tracheostomy. Suction is applied no longer than
   a 5 seconds
   b 5 to 10 seconds
   c 10 seconds
   d 10 to 15 seconds

19 A person's lungs are hyperventilated before suctioning the tracheostomy. Which is used to hyperventilate the lungs?
   a Incentive spirometer
   b Pulse oximeter
   c Ambu bag
   d Partial-rebreathing mask

20 When suctioning a tracheostomy, suction is applied
   a Continuously
   b Intermittently
   c Every 10 seconds
   d As directed by the RN

21 During suction procedures, you can insert the catheter no more than
   a 2 times
   b 3 times
   c 4 times
   d 5 times

22 Mr. Long requires mechanical ventilation. Which is *false?*
   a He has an endotracheal tube or a tracheostomy tube.
   b The call bell must always be within his reach.
   c You should use touch to provide comfort and reassurance.
   d You can reset alarms on the ventilator.

23 An alarm sounds on Mr. Long's ventilator. What should you do first?
   a Reset the alarm.
   b Check to see if his airway is attached to the ventilator.
   c Call the RN immediately.
   d Ask him what is wrong.

24 A person has a pneumothorax. This is the collection of
   a Fluid in the pleural space
   b Blood in the pleural space
   c Air in the pleural space
   d Respiratory secretions in the pleural space

25 A person has chest tubes attached to water-seal drainage. You should do the following *except*
   a Notify the RN if bubbling increases, decreases, or stops
   b Make sure the tubing is not kinked
   c Keep the drainage system below the person's chest
   d Hang tubing in loops

Answers to these questions are on p. 179

5 *Assisting With Urinary Elimination*

OBJECTIVES

- Explain why catheters are used
- Describe the rules for caring for persons with catheters
- Explain the differences between straight and indwelling catheters
- Describe how to collect urine specimens from catheters
- Explain the purpose of bladder irrigations
- Explain how to measure the pH and specific gravity of urine
- Explain how to test urine for blood
- Perform the procedures described in this chapter

KEY TERMS

catheter A tube used to drain or inject fluid through a body opening

catheterization The process of inserting a catheter

dysuria Difficult *(dys)* urination *(uria)*

hematuria Blood *(hemat)* in the urine *(uria)*

irrigation The process of washing out, flushing out, clearing, or cleaning a tube or body cavity

meniscus The curved surface of a column of liquid

residual urine The amount of urine left in the bladder after voiding

This chapter focuses on catheterizations and collecting sterile urine specimens. Measuring urine pH and specific gravity also is presented, along with testing urine for blood. Many hospitals allow assistive personnel to perform these procedures. Before you perform these procedures make sure that:

- Your state allows assistive personnel to perform them
- They are in your job description
- You have the necessary education and training
- You are familiar with the urinary tract structures
- You know how to use the facility's supplies and equipment
- You are comfortable with the procedure
- You review the procedure with an RN
- An RN is available to answer questions and to supervise you

CATHETERIZATIONS

A **catheterization** is the process of inserting a catheter. A **catheter** is a tube used to drain or inject fluid through a body opening. Inserted through the urethra into the bladder, a urinary catheter drains urine. A *straight catheter* drains the bladder and is removed. An *indwelling catheter (retention or Foley catheter)* is left in the bladder so urine drains constantly into a drainage bag. A balloon near the tip is inflated after inserting the catheter. The balloon prevents the catheter from slipping out of the bladder (Fig. 5-1, p. 88). Tubing connects the catheter to the collection bag. The rules listed in Box 5-1 on p. 88 promote the comfort and safety of persons with catheters.

Purpose

Catheters often are inserted before, during, and after surgery to keep the bladder empty. If inserted before or during surgery, the catheter reduces the risk of accidental bladder injury during surgery. After surgery, a full bladder causes pressure on nearby organs. A catheter prevents this problem.

Catheters also allow hourly urinary output measurements in critically ill persons. Catheters are a last resort for incontinence. Catheters do not treat the cause of incontinence, and the risk of infection is high. However, some persons have wounds and pressure sores that need protection from urine. Catheters can protect the wounds and pressure sores from contamination with urine.

Some patients are too weak or disabled to use the bedpan, commode, or toilet. Dying patients are an example. For these patients, catheters can promote comfort. Also, the person is protected from incontinence.

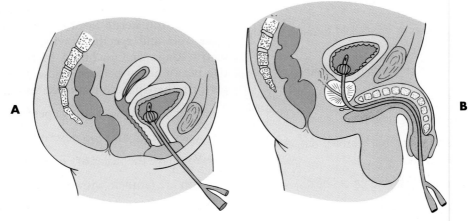

Fig. 5-1 A, *Indwelling catheter in the female bladder. The inflated balloon at the top prevents the catheter from slipping out through the urethra.* **B,** *Indwelling catheter with the balloon inflated in the male bladder.*

BOX 5-1 CARING FOR PERSONS WITH INDWELLING CATHETERS

- Follow the rules of medical asepsis, Standard Precautions, and the Bloodborne Pathogen Standard.

- Make sure urine flows freely through the catheter or tubing. Tubing should not have kinks. The person should not lie on the tubing.

- Keep the drainage bag below the bladder. This prevents urine from flowing backward into the bladder. Attach the drainage bag to the bed frame. *Never attach the drainage bag to the bed rail.* The drainage bag would be higher than the bladder when the bed rail is raised.

- Coil the drainage tubing on the bed. Clamp, tape, or pin it to the bottom linen (Fig. 5-2).

- Secure the catheter to the inner thigh as in Figure 5-2. Or secure it to the man's abdomen. This prevents excessive movement of the catheter and reduces friction at the insertion site. Tape or other devices ordered by the RN are used to secure catheters.

- Check for leaks. Check the site where the catheter connects to the drainage bag. Report any leaks to the RN immediately.

- Provide catheter care if ordered. Catheter care is done daily or twice a day. Some facilities consider perineal care to be sufficient. Catheter care is sometimes needed after bowel movements and when vaginal drainage is present.

- Provide perineal care daily and after bowel movements.

- Empty the drainage bag at the end of the shift or at time intervals as directed by the RN. Also empty it if it becomes full. Measure and record the amount of urine. Report increases or decreases in the amount of urine.

- Use a separate measuring container for each person. This prevents the spread of microbes from one person to another.

- Do not the let the drain on the drainage bag touch any surface.

- Report complaints to the RN immediately. These include complaints of pain, burning, the need to urinate, or irritation. Also report the color, clarity, and odor of urine and the presence of particles.

- Encourage fluid intake as instructed by the RN. ✳

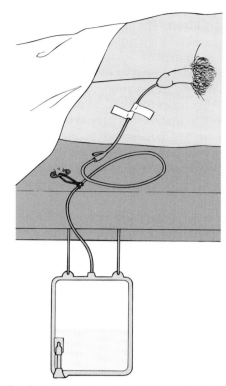

Fig. 5-2 The drainage tubing is coiled on the bed and pinned to the bottom linens so urine flows freely. A rubber band is placed around the tubing with a clove hitch. The safety pin is passed through the loops and pinned to the linens. The catheter is taped to the inner thigh. Enough slack is left on the catheter to prevent friction at the urethra.

Catheters are inserted for diagnostic purposes. They are used to collect sterile urine specimens. Another test involves inserting a catheter to see how much urine is left in the bladder after voiding (**residual urine**). The catheter is inserted right after the person voids.

Straight and Indwelling Catheters

A catheterization requires a doctor's order. The doctor orders a straight catheter or an indwelling catheter. The straight catheter is removed after draining the bladder or obtaining a specimen. An indwelling catheter is left in place and attached to a closed drainage system. A closed drainage system means that nothing can enter the system from the catheter to the drainage bag.

Catheterizations require sterile technique (see Chapter 2). The urinary system is sterile. Catheterizations increase the risk of urinary tract infections (UTI). These are common nosocomial (facility acquired) infections. These infections prolong the person's recovery. They are costly to treat. Some cause life-threatening complications. Older persons are at risk (see Focus on Older Persons, p. 90). So are women. The distance from the meatus (urethral opening) and the bladder is shorter in women than in men. Therefore microbes have a shorter distance to travel in women than in men. Also, the meatus is close to the vagina and to the anus. These areas are not sterile and contain microbes that can easily enter the urinary system. Contaminating the sterile field, catheter, or other supplies increases the risk of a UTI. Contamination occurs easily during a catheterization. You must be very careful.

Equipment and supplies The RN tells you what size catheter to use, what kind of catheter to use (straight or indwelling), and if a closed drainage system is needed. With this information, you select a straight or indwelling catheterization kit from the supply area. The kit has supplies for the procedure. All items in the kit are sterile. The kit usually contains:

- The catheter
- Sterile gloves
- Sterile drape for under the buttocks (female) or across the thighs (male)
- Fenestrated drape (*fenestrated* means with an opening or window) for the perineal area
- Forceps
- Basin for urine
- Lubricant
- Antiseptic solution
- Cotton balls
- Syringe with sterile water (see p. 99)
- Drainage bag and tubing (indwelling catheter kit)
- Plastic clamp

Catheters are sized in the French scale. (The abbreviation "Fr" means French.) Either *Fr* follows the number or the # sign is before the number. The RN tells you what size to use. The following are guidelines:

- Children—6, 8, or 10 Fr (#6, #8, or #10)
- Women—14 or 16 Fr (#14 or #16)
- Men—14, 16, or 18 Fr (#14, #16, or #18)

Good lighting is essential for the procedure. A flashlight or gooseneck lamp helps you see the urinary meatus. Place the light source at the foot of the bed, and direct it at the perineal area.

Types of catheters A straight catheter (Fig. 5-3, *A*, p. 90) has one lumen (passageway). An indwelling catheter has a double lumen (Fig. 5-3, *B*, p. 90). Sterile water is injected

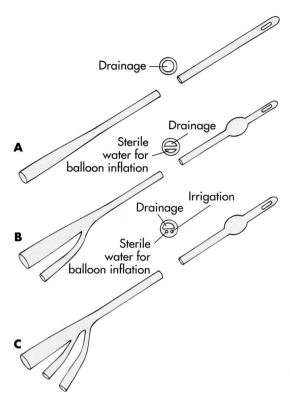

Fig. 5-3 *Types of catheters.* **A,** *Straight catheter (single lumen).* **B,** *Indwelling catheter (double lumen) with balloon inflated.* **C,** *Indwelling catheter with a triple-lumen catheter. The balloon is inflated.*

through one lumen to inflate the balloon. Urine drains from the bladder through the other lumen. Some indwelling catheters are triple lumen (Fig. 5-3, *C*). The third lumen is for bladder treatments ordered by the doctor.

Preparing the Person

The RN explains the procedure and its need to the person. The RN also explains the care required while the catheter is in place. This helps the person understand what is happening and why. You explain the procedure before beginning. During the procedure, explain to the person what you are doing step by step. This information helps meet the person's need for safety and security. The informed person is likely to be more relaxed and cooperative.

The procedure is embarrassing for some people. It involves exposing and touching the genitals. The person needs to know how privacy is protected during the procedure. Explain that you will draw the privacy curtain, close window shades or drapes, and close room doors. Also explain how draping is done and that the perineal area is exposed only for a short time. If the procedure embarrasses you, share your feelings with the RN.

focus on children The child may not be cooperative. Although the child may not understand the procedure, you still need to explain what you are going to do. You are likely to need a parent or co-worker to help keep the child in position. Restricting the child's movement is likely to further upset the child. However, the child needs to be kept still so that the sterile field is not contaminated.

Adolescents are concerned about genital development. They are likely to be embarrassed about having someone look at and touch the perineal area. You need to thoroughly explain what you are going to do. A professional manner is important.

Adolescent boys may have an erection when the genitals are touched. If this happens, give him privacy. Cover the area, and tell the boy you will give him some time alone. Tell him when you will return, and leave the room. Close the door as you leave the room, and knock on the door when you return. (This applies to adolescent boys and adult men of all ages.)

focus on older persons When catheterizing women, they are positioned as for perineal care. Older women may not be able to hold the position. You need a co-worker to help the patient maintain the position. Work as quickly as you can to complete the procedure.

If possible, catheterizations are avoided in elderly persons because of the risk of UTIs. Changes in the urinary system from aging increase the older person's risk for UTIs. These infections are especially serious for elderly persons. They can lead to serious health problems and death.

Enlargement of the prostate gland is a common problem in older men. The gland lies just below the bladder. When the gland enlarges, it can obstruct the urethra. Urine does not flow out of the bladder normally. The urine stream is less forceful. The bladder does not empty completely. Dribbling, frequent urination, and nocturia (urination at night) are common problems. Catheterization is sometimes necessary. A Coudé catheter is often used. It has a curved tip and is easier to pass around the obstruction. Because of the obstruction, a doctor or RN inserts the Coudé catheter.

focus on home care Make sure an RN is available by phone in case problems arise. Remember that you cannot pick up the phone and dial with sterile gloves. Nor can you answer the phone. When you review the procedure with the RN, ask what you should do if problems occur.

Text continued on p. 96

PRE-PROCEDURE

1 Explain the procedure to the person.

2 Collect the following:

- Catheterization kit as directed by the RN; check the kit for needed supplies (see p. 89)
- Sterile gloves (if not part of the kit)
- Flashlight or gooseneck lamp
- Bath blanket
- Soap
- Bath basin with warm water
- Washcloth
- Towel
- Disposable gloves
- Specimen container and laboratory requisition (if ordered)
- Leakproof bag

3 Identify the person. Check the ID bracelet with the assignment sheet.

4 Provide for privacy.

5 Raise the bed to the best level for good body mechanics. Make sure the far bed rail is raised.

PROCEDURE

6 Position the person supine. Cover the person with a bath blanket.

7 Position and drape the person as for perineal care.

8 Put on the disposable gloves.

9 Provide perineal care.

10 Remove equipment and supplies used for perineal care. Also remove the gloves and wash your hands. (Make sure both bed rails are up when you leave the bedside. Lower the near bed rail when you return.)

11 Position the flashlight or gooseneck lamp at the foot of the bed. Direct the light source at the perineal area.

12 Arrange the overbed table and catheterization kit so you can create a sterile field.

13 Place the leakproof bag in a convenient location.

14 Open the catheterization kit. Follow directions on the package.

15 Put on the sterile gloves.

16 Organize the sterile field:

a Open sterile packages and containers (cotton balls, antiseptic solution, specimen container, and lubricant).

b Pour the antiseptic solution over the cotton balls.

17 Pick up the first sterile drape. Stand back, and allow it to unfold.

18 Drape the person:

a Draping a female:

1) Hold the drape with both hands.

2) Do not touch her or the bed with your gloves. Your gloves must touch only the sterile drape.

3) Ask the woman to raise her buttocks off the bed.

4) Slide the drape under her buttocks.

5) Pick up the fenestrated drape, and let it unfold.

6) Drape it over the perineum. Expose only the labia.

b Draping a male:

1) Lift the penis with your nondominant hand. (This hand is now contaminated. It cannot touch any part of the sterile field.)

2) Lay the drape over the thighs.

3) Pick up the fenestrated drape with your sterile hand. Let it unfold.

4) Position the drape over the penis.

5) Lift the penis through the opening in the drape with your contaminated hand. Lay the penis on the drape.

19 Place the catheterization tray and its contents on the drape between the person's legs.

20 Lubricate the catheter:

a Female: lubricate about 1 to 2 inches (2.5 to 5 cm) of the catheter tip.

b Male: lubricate about 3 to 5 inches (7.5 to 12.5 cm) of the catheter tip.

Continued

INSERTING A STRAIGHT CATHETER—CONT'D

PROCEDURE—CONT'D

21 Clean the meatus with the cotton balls. Pick them up with the forceps. Use a sterile cotton ball for each stroke. (Discard used cotton balls into the trash bag. Do not let the forceps touch the bag.)

  a Female (Fig. 5-4, p. 94):

    1) Separate the labia majora with the thumb and index finger of your nondominant hand. (This hand is now contaminated and cannot touch any part of the sterile field.)

    2) Keep the labia separated until you insert the catheter.

    3) Use your sterile hand to pick up the forceps.

    4) Pick up a cotton ball with the forceps.

    5) Clean the labia minora on the side away from you. Wipe from the clitoris to the anus with one stroke. Discard the cotton ball.

    6) Clean the labia minora on the side near you. Wipe from the clitoris to the anus with one stroke. Discard the cotton ball.

    7) Clean the meatus. Wipe from the top down. Discard the cotton ball.

  b Male:

    1) Pick up the penis with your contaminated hand.

    2) Retract the foreskin if the man is not circumcised (Fig. 5-5, p. 94).

    3) Hold the penis firmly behind the glans as in Figure 5-6 on p. 94. Maintain this position until you insert the catheter.

    4) Pick up a cotton ball using the sterile forceps.

    5) Clean the penis starting at the meatus. Use a circular motion. Discard the cotton ball.

    6) Wipe around the meatus using a circular motion. Discard the cotton ball.

    7) Clean to where your fingers are holding the penis. Discard the cotton ball.

22 Place the drainage end of the catheter into the collecting basin.

23 Pick up the catheter about 2 inches from the tip. Make sure the drainage end stays in the collecting basin.

24 Insert the catheter (Fig. 5-7, p. 94):

  a Female:

    1) Make sure you can see the meatus. Also locate the vaginal opening.

    2) Ask the person to take a deep breath.

    3) Insert the catheter into the meatus until urine flows (about 3 inches). Insert gently and slowly. (Do not push the catheter if you feel resistance. Stop the procedure and call for the RN.)

    4) Hold the catheter in place with your contaminated hand.

    5) If no urine flows, the catheter could be in the vagina. Leave the catheter in place, and get a new catheterization kit. Begin at step 14. If a co-worker is with you, ask that person to get you another catheter. Keep the labia retracted. Have the co-worker peel back the packaging so that you can grasp the catheter. Lubricate the catheter, and insert it. Remove the catheter from the vagina when urine flows.

INSERTING A STRAIGHT CATHETER—CONT'D

PROCEDURE—CONT'D

b Male:

   1) Hold the penis so it is upright as in Fig. 5-6.

   2) Ask the person to bear down as if voiding.

   3) Insert the catheter into the meatus.

   4) Advance the catheter until urine flows (about 8 inches).

   5) Lay the penis on the drape. Hold the catheter in place with your contaminated hand.

   6) Do not force the catheter if you feel resistance. Stop the procedure, and call for the RN.

25 Collect a urine specimen if ordered. Continue to hold the catheter in place with your contaminated hand:

   a Hold the end of the catheter over the specimen container with your sterile hand. Collect about 30 ml of urine.

   b Pinch the catheter to stop urine flow.

   c Cover the specimen container, and set it aside.

26 Place the end of the catheter into the collecting basin.

27 Let the bladder empty according to the RN's instructions. Facility policy may require you to stop urine flow for 15 to 20 minutes after draining 750 to 1000 ml. (Rapid emptying can cause the person to go into shock.)

28 Note the amount of urine collected.

29 Remove the catheter slowly.

30 Return foreskin to its natural position.

31 Remove and discard the gloves. Gather equipment and supplies for disposal.

32 Cover the person, and remove the bath blanket.

33 Thank the person for cooperating.

POST-PROCEDURE

34 Make sure the person is comfortable.

35 Raise or lower bed rails as instructed by the RN.

36 Lower the bed to its lowest position.

37 Place the call bell within reach.

38 Clean the wash basin. Return reusable supplies to their proper place.

39 Wipe off the overbed table.

40 Unscreen the person.

41 Follow facility policy for dirty linen.

42 Wash your hands.

43 Report your observations to the RN:

- The amount of urine obtained
- Color, clarity, and odor of urine
- Any particles in the urine
- How the person tolerated the procedure
- Any other observation

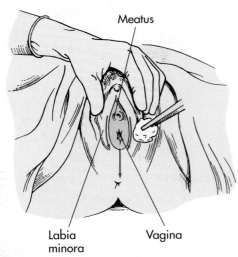

Fig. 5-4 *Cleaning the female meatus. Clean from top to bottom using a sterile cotton ball for each stroke.* (From Potter PA, Perry AG: Fundamentals of nursing: concepts, process, and practice, *ed 4, St Louis, 1997, Mosby.)*

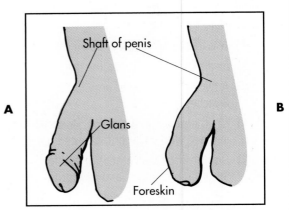

Fig. 5-5 *A, Circumcised male. B, Uncircumcised male.*

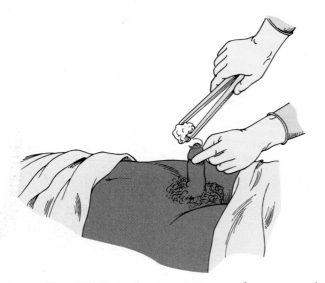

Fig. 5-6 *Cleaning the male meatus. Start at the meatus using circular motions. Clean downward to your fingers. Use a sterile cotton ball for each stroke.* (From Potter PA, Perry AG: Fundamentals of nursing: concepts, process, and practice, *ed 4, St Louis, 1997, Mosby.)*

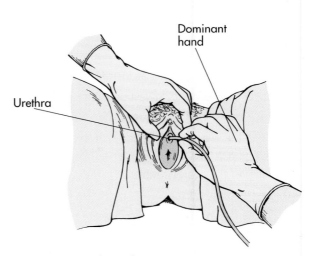

Fig. 5-7 *Inserting the catheter.* (From Potter PA, Perry AG: Fundamentals of nursing: concepts, process, and practice, *ed 4, St Louis, 1997, Mosby.)*

INSERTING AN INDWELLING CATHETER

PRE-PROCEDURE

1 Explain the procedure to the person.

2 Collect equipment:
   - Catheterization kit as directed by the RN (see p. 89).
   - Flashlight or gooseneck lamp
   - Bath blanket
   - Soap
   - Bath basin with warm water
   - Washcloth
   - Towel
   - Disposable gloves
   - Trash bag
   - Nonallergenic tape
   - Safety pin and rubber band (optional)

3 Identify the person. Check the ID bracelet with the assignment sheet.

4 Provide for privacy.

5 Raise the bed to the best level for good body mechanics. Make sure the far bed rail is raised.

PROCEDURE

6 Follow steps 6 through 16 in *Inserting a Straight Catheter*.

7 Make sure the catheter is attached to the collecting tubing and the drainage container. Make sure the drain is closed.

8 Test the balloon on the indwelling catheter (Fig. 5-8, p. 96). It must inflate and not leak:
   a Attach the prefilled syringe to the balloon valve.
   b Inject the water. The balloon should inflate.
   c Pull back on the syringe to withdraw the fluid.
   d Leave the syringe attached to the balloon port.

9 Drape the person as in *Inserting a Straight Catheter*, steps 17 and 18.

10 Place the sterile catheterization tray and its contents on the drape between the person's legs.

11 Lubricate the catheter.

12 Clean the meatus.

13 Insert the catheter until urine appears.

14 Female: advance the catheter another 2 inches after urine appears.

   Male: advance the catheter another 2 or 3 inches after urine appears. (Check facility policy. Some facilities require advancing the catheter farther. This is done to make sure the balloon is inflated in the bladder, not in the urethra [see Step 16].)

15 Hold the catheter in place with your nondominant hand.

16 Inflate the balloon. Inject the contents of the syringe. (Pull back on the syringe to withdraw the water if the person complains of pain or discomfort. Insert the catheter farther. Inject fluid again.)

17 Remove the syringe.

18 Let go of the catheter with your nondominant hand. Return foreskin to its natural position.

19 Pull on the catheter gently. You should feel resistance. Resistance means that the balloon is holding the catheter in place (see Fig. 5-1).

Continued

INSERTING AN INDWELLING CATHETER—CONT'D

PROCEDURE—CONT'D

20 Secure the catheter in place. Allow enough slack so there is no pull on the catheter:

   a Female: tape the catheter to the inner thigh.

   b Male: tape the catheter to the top of the thigh or lower abdomen.

21 Secure the drainage container to the bed frame.

22 Coil tubing on the bed as in Figure 5-2. Clamp, pin, or tape the tubing to the bottom sheet.

23 Remove and discard the gloves. Gather equipment and supplies for disposal.

24 Cover the person, and remove the bath blanket.

25 Thank the person for cooperating.

POST-PROCEDURE

26 Follow steps 34 through 43 in *Inserting a Straight Catheter.*

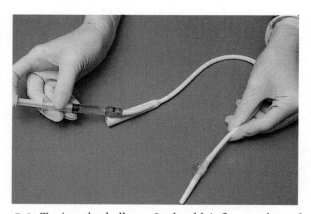

Fig. 5-8 *Testing the balloon. It should inflate and not leak.* *(From Potter PA, Perry AG:* Fundamentals of nursing: concepts, process, and practice, *ed 4, St Louis, 1997, Mosby.)*

REMOVING INDWELLING CATHETERS

The doctor gives the order to remove the catheter. Some persons need bladder training before the catheter is removed. Dysuria and frequency are common problems after removing catheters. **Dysuria** means difficult *(dys)* urination *(uria).*

Removing an indwelling catheter involves deflating the balloon. You need a syringe large enough to hold the balloon's contents. Check the label at the end of the catheter for balloon size. The RN also tells you what size syringe to use.

The RN tells you when to remove a catheter. Make sure you review the procedure with the RN. Also, practice Standard Precautions and follow the Bloodborne Pathogen Standard.

REMOVING AN INDWELLING CATHETER

PRE-PROCEDURE

1 Explain the procedure to the person.
2 Wash your hands.
3 Collect the following:
   - Disposable towel
   - Syringe as directed by the RN
   - Trash receptacle
   - Gloves (nonsterile)
   - Bath blanket
4 Identify the person. Check the ID bracelet with the assignment sheet.
5 Provide for privacy.
6 Raise the bed to the best level for body mechanics. Make sure the far bed rail is raised.

PROCEDURE

7 Position the person as for a catheterization.
8 Drape the person with a bath blanket.
9 Put on the gloves.
10 Remove the tape securing the catheter to the person.
11 Place the towel:
   a Female: between her legs
   b Male: over his thighs
12 Attach the syringe to the balloon port.
13 Pull back on the syringe slowly to withdraw all the water from the balloon. For example, if the balloon is 5 ml, you should withdraw 5 ml into the syringe. Call for the RN if you cannot remove all the water.
14 Withdraw the catheter gently. Do not withdraw the catheter while water is in the balloon.
15 Place the catheter in the trash receptacle.
16 Dry the perineal area with the towel.
17 Remove the gloves.
18 Cover the person, and remove the bath blanket. Make sure the person is comfortable.
19 Raise bed rails as instructed by the RN.
20 Lower the bed to its lowest position.
21 Place the call bell within reach.

POST-PROCEDURE

22 Put on gloves.
23 Take the drainage container to the bathroom.
24 Measure the amount of urine in the drainage bag. Note the amount.
25 Discard the urine.
26 Place the drainage bag in trash container. Or discard the drainage bag following facility policy.
27 Remove and discard the gloves.
28 Wash your hands.
29 Report your observations to the RN (see p. 93).

BLADDER IRRIGATIONS

An **irrigation** is the process of washing out, flushing out, clearing, or cleaning a tube or body cavity. Water, saline, or medicated solutions are used depending on the purpose and site of the irrigation. *Bladder irrigations* are done to wash out the bladder or to treat bladder infections. The doctor orders the procedure, the required solution, and the amount of solution. Sterile technique is required.

Bladder irrigations usually involve sterile saline or a medicated solution. A common irrigation procedure involves a triple lumen catheter (Fig. 5-9). The irrigation bag is attached to one lumen and the drainage bag to another. The third lumen is for inflating the catheter balloon. The irrigation bag hangs from an IV pole. Solution flows into the bladder through the irrigation lumen in the catheter. It drains, along with urine, from the bladder through the drainage lumen in the catheter. The solution and urine collect in the drainage bag.

To measure urine output, the RN notes the amount of irrigating solution used. This amount is subtracted from the amount of fluid in the collection bag. The remaining amount is urine. For example, 1000 ml of irrigation solution was used. The drainage bag contained 1450 ml of fluid. Subtracting 1000 ml from 1450 ml leaves 450 ml of urine:

$$\begin{array}{r} 1450 \text{ ml (solution and urine)} \\ - 1000 \text{ ml (solution)} \\ \hline 450 \text{ ml (urine)} \end{array}$$

A bladder irrigation is done by RNs and LPNs/LVNs. You may be asked to assist. Some states and facilities let assistive personnel perform the procedure. If assistive personnel are allowed to do the procedure, the facility will provide the necessary education and training.

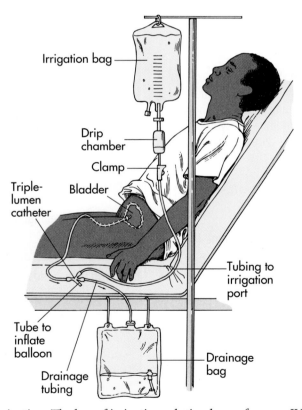

Fig. 5-9 *Bladder irrigation. The bag of irrigating solution hangs from an IV pole. The irrigating solution flows into the bladder through the irrigation port in the catheter. The solution and urine drain out of the bladder through the catheter's drainage port. The solution and urine collect in the drainage bag.* (*From Potter PA, Perry AG:* Fundamentals of nursing: concepts, process, and practice, *ed 4, St Louis, 1997, Mosby.*)

THE STERILE URINE SPECIMEN

With a closed drainage system, nothing can enter the system from the catheter to the drainage bag. You cannot disconnect the catheter from the drainage tubing to collect a specimen. Otherwise microbes enter the system. Nor can you collect a specimen from the drainage bag. The drainage bag is an environment that promotes the growth of microbes. To collect a specimen, urine is withdrawn from the catheter under sterile conditions. A sterile needle and syringe are used. Microbes do not enter the system with sterile technique.

The catheter must be self-sealing or have a collection port. Rubber catheters are self-sealing. Plastic, silicone, or Silastic catheters are not. The RN tells you when to collect a sterile urine specimen and what type of catheter the person has.

Handling Syringes and Needles

Syringes are made of plastic. A syringe has three parts (Fig. 5-10): tip, barrel, and plunger. The needle attaches to the tip. The outside of the barrel is marked to show amounts. The inside of the barrel is for fluid. You use the plunger to inject or withdraw fluid. When you push the plunger in, fluid is injected. To withdraw fluid, pull the plunger back. The tip, inside of the barrel, and plunger shaft are sterile. You can touch only the outside of the barrel and the top of the plunger.

Needles are made of stainless steel. A needle has three parts (see Fig. 5-10): hub, shaft, and bevel. The hub attaches to the syringe tip. The shaft varies in length ($\frac{1}{4}$ to 5 inches) and gauge (diameter). Needle gauges vary from #14 to #28. The smaller the gauge number, the larger the needle diameter. The bevel (sharp part of the needle) is slanted. Bevels are short or long. Needles are sterile. You cannot touch any part of the needle. A needle cover caps the needle to prevent contamination or needle stick injuries.

Sterile syringes and needles are packaged together or separately in peel-back packaging (see p. 26). If separate, attach the capped needle to the syringe tip. To use the syringe and needle, pull the cap straight off the needle. *After use, discard the needle and syringe into a sharps disposable container. Do not remove the needle from the syringe. Do not recap the needle. Do not bend or break the needle. Follow Standard Precautions and the Bloodborne Pathogen Standard when using needles.*

The RN tells you what size syringe and needle to use. Depending on the test, a 3-ml or 30-ml syringe is used. Small-gauge needles (#23 or #25) are usually used. Large-gauge needles can leave holes in the catheter or collection port.

Text continued on p. 102

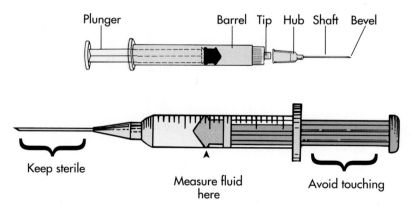

Fig. 5-10 *Parts of syringe and needle. Note that the needle, plunger shaft, and inside of the barrel are sterile. (Modified from Potter PA, Perry AG:* Fundamentals of nursing: concepts, process, and practice, *ed 4, St Louis, 1997, Mosby.)*

COLLECTING A STERILE URINE SPECIMEN FROM AN INDWELLING CATHETER

PRE-PROCEDURE

1 Explain the procedure to the person.

2 Wash your hands.

3 Put on gloves (nonsterile).

4 Clamp the drainage tube for 15 to 30 minutes as directed by the RN (Fig. 5-11). This lets urine collect in the catheter. (Provide privacy during this step.)

5 Remove the gloves, and wash your hands.

6 Collect the following:
- Syringe and needle as directed by the RN
- Antiseptic swabs
- Sterile specimen container
- Label
- Plastic bag
- Gloves

7 Provide for privacy.

PROCEDURE

8 Label the specimen container.

9 Identify the person. Check the ID bracelet with the requisition slip.

10 Put on gloves.

11 Open the specimen container. Set the container and lid in a convenient location. Set the lid down so the inside is up.

12 Expose the catheter site.

13 Clean the puncture site with an antiseptic swab. Use the collection port or end of a self-sealing catheter (just above where the catheter connects to the drainage tubing).

14 Unclamp the catheter.

15 Remove the needle cap. Pull the cap straight off the needle.

16 Insert the needle at a 90-degree angle into a collection port (Fig. 5-12). Insert the needle at a 30-degree angle into a self-sealing catheter (Fig. 5-13). Insert the needle carefully so that it does not go all the way through the catheter and out the other side.

17 Pull back on the plunger to fill the syringe with urine.

18 Transfer syringe contents into the specimen container. Push down on the plunger to eject urine from the syringe. The needle must not touch the outside of the specimen container.

19 Put the lid on the specimen container. Place the container in a plastic bag.

20 Discard the syringe and needle into a sharps disposable container.

21 Unclamp the tubing. Make sure urine flows into the drainage bag.

22 Cover the person.

23 Remove the gloves.

POST-PROCEDURE

24 Make sure the person is comfortable.

25 Place the call bell within reach.

26 Unscreen the person.

27 Discard disposable supplies.

28 Wash your hands.

29 Report your observations to the RN.

30 Take the urine specimen and laboratory requisition slip to the laboratory.

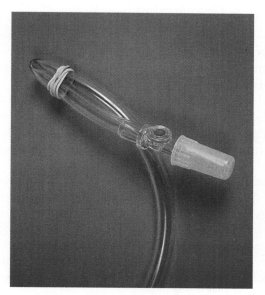

Fig. 5-11 *Catheter tubing is clamped with a rubber band.* *(From Elkin MK, Perry AG, Potter PA:* Nursing interventions and clinical skills, *St Louis, 1996, Mosby.)*

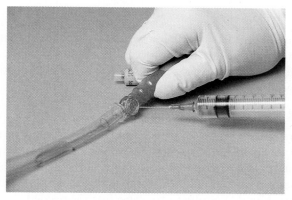

Fig. 5-12 *The needle is inserted at a 90-degree angle into the collection port. (From Elkin MK, Perry AG, Potter PA:* Nursing interventions and clinical skills, *St Louis, 1996, Mosby.)*

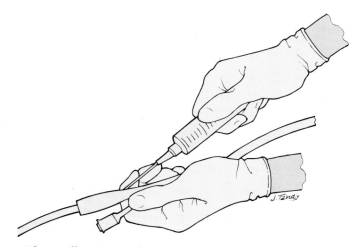

Fig. 5-13 *The needle is inserted at a 30-degree angle into a self-sealing catheter.*

TESTING URINE

The RN may ask you to do simple urine tests. You can test pH and for the presence of blood using reagent strips. You also can test specific gravity.

Testing pH

Urine pH measures if urine is acidic or alkaline. Changes in normal pH (4.6 to 8.0) occur from illness, foods, and medications. Use reagent strips to test urine pH. A routine urine specimen is needed.

Testing for Blood

Normal urine is free of blood. Injury and disease can cause blood *(hemat)* to appear in the urine *(uria)*. This is called **hematuria.** Sometimes blood is seen in the urine. At other times it is unseen *(occult)*. You use reagent strips to test for occult blood. A routine urine specimen is needed.

Using reagent strips Reagent strips have different sections that change color when they react with urine. To use a reagent strip, dip the strip into urine. Then compare the strip with the color chart on the bottle. The RN gives you specific instructions for the urine test ordered. You must read the manufacturer's instructions before you begin.

Measuring Specific Gravity

Urine contains particles and dissolved solids. Urine specific gravity measures the amount of these substances in comparison with water. When urine contains large amounts of particles and dissolved solids, urine is concentrated. The amount of water is less than normal, and the amount of substances is higher than normal. Concentrated urine is dark yellow. Specific gravity is high. Dilute urine contains large amounts of water and few substances. Urine is pale, and specific gravity is low.

A *urinometer* measures *(meter)* the specific gravity of urine *(urino)*. This device has two parts (Fig. 5-14). The scale is calibrated in 0.001 units. The scale ranges from 1.000 to 1.060. The bottom part is a mercury-filled bulb. This part gives the urinometer weight. To measure specific gravity, the urinometer is placed in a cylinder of urine. The urinometer sinks into the urine and floats as in Figure 5-14.

Normal specific gravity is between 1.010 and 1.035. Place the urinometer at eye level to read the measurement. Read the measurement at the base of the **meniscus** of urine. (A meniscus is the curved surface of a column of liquid.)

Refractometers (Fig. 5-15) are used by laboratory personnel to test urine for specific gravity. A drop of urine is placed on the prism. The refractometer is held toward light. Then the measurement is read.

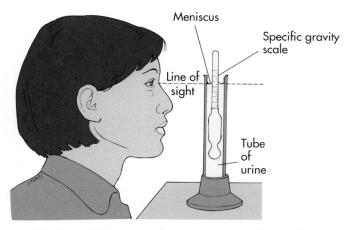

Fig. 5-14 *Urinometer for measuring specific gravity.*

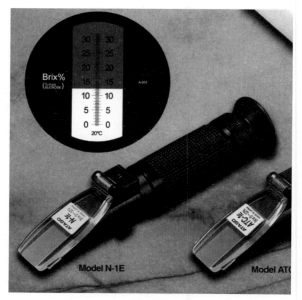

Fig. 5-15 *Refractometer measures specific gravity.* *(From MSDivisions.)*

MEASURING SPECIFIC GRAVITY

PRE-PROCEDURE

1 Explain the procedure to the person.
2 Wash your hands.
3 Collect a urinometer and gloves.

4 Identify the person. Check the ID bracelet with the assignment sheet.
5 Provide for privacy.

PROCEDURE

6 Put on the gloves.
7 Collect a urine specimen as directed by the RN.
8 Fill the glass cylinder about ¾ full (about 20 ml) with urine.
9 Place the urinometer in the cylinder.
10 Spin the urinometer between your thumb and index finger. Spin the urinometer again if it stops against the cylinder. The urinometer should float freely.

11 Place the urinometer at eye level.
12 Read the measurement at the base of the meniscus. Note the measurement.
13 Discard the urine, and clean the urinometer.
14 Clean the bedpan, urinal, or specimen pan.
15 Return equipment to its proper place.
16 Remove the gloves.
17 Help the person wash the hands.

POST-PROCEDURE

18 Make sure the person is comfortable.
19 Place the call bell within reach.
20 Raise or lower bed rails as instructed by the RN.

21 Unscreen the person.
22 Wash your hands.
23 Report your observations to the RN.

SUMMARY

Catheterizations are sterile procedures. Surgical asepsis is practiced to prevent microbes from entering the sterile urinary system. Catheterizations increase the risk of urinary tract infections. These infections are serious. They increase the cost and length of recovery. For older persons, UTIs can lead to death.

You must not contaminate equipment, supplies, or the sterile field when catheterizing a person. If you do contaminate, be honest with yourself and the RN. Correct the situation, and restart the procedure.

Starting over with sterile items is easier and cheaper than treating a UTI.

Specific gravity, pH, and testing urine for blood all require accurate measurements. The doctor uses the test results for diagnosing and prescribing treatments. Your measurements affect the doctor's decisions. Accurate measurements benefit the patient. Inaccurate measurements place the patient at risk for the wrong diagnosis and treatment. Be careful and honest when testing urine.

REVIEW QUESTIONS

Circle the best *answer.*

1 Catheterizations are done for these reasons *except*
   a Diagnosing
   b Staff convenience when a person needs to urinate often
   c To keep the bladder empty during and after surgery
   d To protect wounds and pressure sores from urine contamination

2 Catheterizations increase the risk of
   a High specific gravity
   b Blood in the urine
   c Urinary tract infection
   d Low pH

3 A person has an indwelling catheter. Which is *incorrect?*
   a Keep the drainage bag above the level of the bladder.
   b Make sure the drainage tubing is free of kinks.
   c Coil the drainage tubing on the bed.
   d Tape the catheter to the inner thigh.

4 A person has an indwelling catheter. Which is *false?*
   a Tape any leaks at the connection site.
   b Follow the rules of medical asepsis and Standard Precautions.
   c Empty the drainage bag at the end of each shift.
   d Report complaints of pain, burning, the need to urinate, or irritation immediately.

5 You are going to catheterize Mr. Clark. You need the following information from the RN *except*
   a If a straight or indwelling catheter was ordered
   b What size catheter to use
   c What size needle to use
   d If a urine specimen is needed

6 A catheterization requires
   a Sterile technique
   b Medical asepsis
   c A closed drainage system
   d Perineal care after the procedure

7 You are inserting a straight catheter. Which is part of the procedure?
   a Attaching the catheter to a closed drainage system
   b Testing the balloon before inserting the catheter
   c Letting the bladder empty
   d Tugging gently on the catheter to make sure it is in place

8 You are going to remove an indwelling catheter. You
   a Attach a needle to a syringe
   b Check the size of the balloon
   c Tug on the catheter to make sure it is in place
   d Use an alcohol swab to clean the site

9 You are going to remove a catheter with a 5-ml balloon. You withdraw only 3 ml. What should you do?
   a Call for the RN.
   b Inject the fluid.
   c Pull out the catheter gently.
   d Make sure the needle is attached to the syringe.

REVIEW QUESTIONS—CONT'D

10 You are going to obtain a sterile urine specimen from an indwelling catheter. You need to use a needle and syringe. Which is *false?*

a The tip, inside of the barrel, and plunger shaft of the syringe are sterile.

b The needle is sterile. You cannot touch the hub, shaft, or bevel.

c You can touch the top of the plunger and the outside barrel.

d The needle is recapped after obtaining the urine specimen.

11 Urine is tested for blood and pH using

a Reagent strips

b A urinometer

c A sterile urine specimen

d A meniscus

12 When the specific gravity is low, the urine

a Is pale

b Contains blood

c Is contaminated

d Is tested with reagent strips

Answers to these questions are on p. 179

6 Assisting With Enteral Nutrition

KEY TERMS

aspiration The breathing of fluid or an object into the lungs

enteral nutrition Giving nutrients through the gastrointestinal tract *(enteral)*

gastrostomy An opening *(stomy)* into the stomach *(gastro)*

jejunostomy An opening *(stomy)* into the middle part of the small intestine *(jejuno)*

nasogastric (NG) tube A tube inserted through the nose *(naso)* into the stomach *(gastro)*

nasointestinal tube A tube inserted through the nose into the duodenum or jejunum of the small intestine

percutaneous endoscopic gastrostomy (PEG) tube A tube inserted into the stomach *(gastro)* through a stab or puncture wound *(stomy)* made through *(per)* the skin *(cutaneous)*; a lighted instrument *(scope)* allows the doctor to see inside a body cavity or organ *(endo)*

regurgitation The backward flow of food from the stomach into the mouth

Persons who cannot chew or swallow often require enteral nutrition. **Enteral nutrition** is giving nutrients through the gastrointestinal tract *(enteral)*. Formula is given through a feeding tube inserted into the stomach or small intestine:

- A **nasogastric (NG) tube** is inserted through the nose *(naso)* into the stomach *(gastro)* (Fig. 6-1). A doctor or an RN performs the procedure.

- A **nasointestinal tube** is inserted through the nose into the duodenum or jejunum of the small intestine (Fig. 6-2, p. 108). A doctor or an RN performs the procedure.

- A **gastrostomy** is an opening *(stomy)* into the stomach *(gastro)* (Fig. 6-3, p. 108). The opening is created surgically.

- A **jejunostomy** is an opening *(stomy)* into the middle part of the small intestine *(jejuno)* (Fig. 6-4, p. 108). The opening is created surgically.

- A **percutaneous endoscopic gastrostomy (PEG) tube** is inserted with an endoscope. An endoscope is a lighted instrument *(scope)*. It allows the doctor to see inside a body cavity or organ *(endo)*. The endoscope allows the doctor to see inside the stomach. The doctor inserts the endoscope through the person's mouth and esophagus and into the stomach. A stab or puncture wound *(stomy)* is made through *(per)* the skin *(cutaneous)* and into the stomach *(gastro)*. A tube is inserted into the stomach through the stab wound (Fig. 6-5, p. 109).

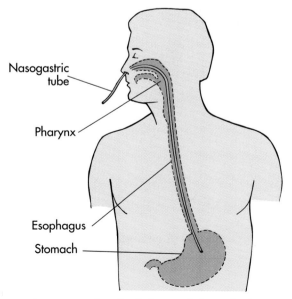

Fig. 6-1 *A nasogastric tube is inserted through the nose and esophagus into the stomach.*

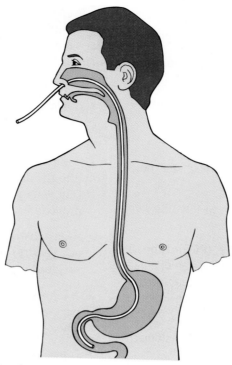

Fig. 6-2 *A nasointestinal tube is inserted through the nose into the duodenum or jejunum of the small intestine.*

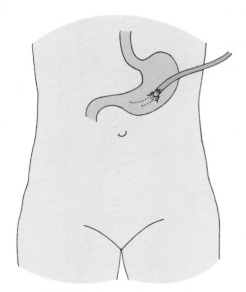

Fig. 6-3 *A gastrostomy tube.*

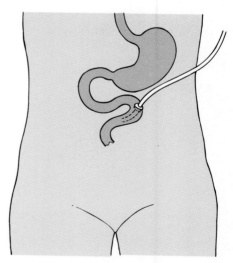

Fig. 6-4 *A jejunostomy tube.*

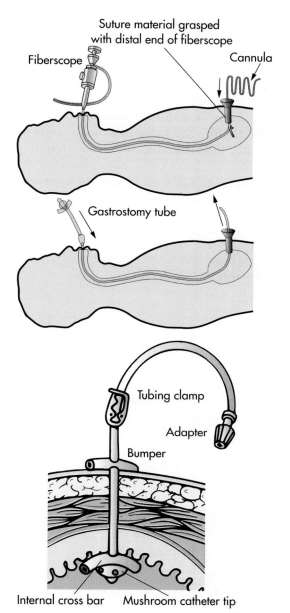

Fig. 6-5 *A percutaneous endoscopic gastrostomy. (From Lewis SM, Collier IC, Heitkemper MM:* Medical-surgical nursing: assessment and management of clinical problems, *ed 4, St Louis, 1996, Mosby.)*

PURPOSE

Feeding tubes are used when food cannot pass normally from the mouth into the esophagus and then into the stomach. Cancer of the head, neck, or esophagus is a common cause. So is trauma or surgery to the face, mouth, head, or neck. Coma is another reason for tube feedings. Some persons with dementia no longer know how to eat and may require tube feedings. Gastrostomy, jejunostomy, and PEG feedings are used for long-term enteral nutrition. The ostomy may be temporary or permanent.

FORMULAS

The doctor orders the type of formula and the amount to give. Most formulas contain protein, carbohydrates, fat, vitamins, and minerals. Commercial formulas are common. Sometimes formula is prepared by the dietary department.

Formulas provide an environment for the growth of microorganisms. Contamination can occur when preparing, storing, or giving tube feedings. To prevent contamination:

- Wear gloves when preparing or handling formula. Replace soiled gloves as necessary.

- Do not use dented or damaged cans.

- Check the expiration date on commercial formulas. Return expired products to the supply area.

- Check the date on formulas prepared by the dietary department. Discard any formula more than 24 hours old.

- Wash cans or bottles before opening them.

- Label cans or bottles with the time and date opened.

- Refrigerate open cans or prepared formula. Place a tight cover or lid over the container. Use the formula within 24 hours. Discard formula more than 24 hours old.

- Clear the tube before and after the feeding. Use 30 to 50 ml of water or other fluid according to facility policy. (This is part of the person's intake. Total intake for a feeding is often limited to 450 ml.)

SCHEDULED AND CONTINUOUS FEEDINGS

The doctor orders scheduled or continuous feedings. Scheduled feedings usually are given four times a day with a syringe or feeding bag (Fig. 6-6). Usually about 400 ml is given over 20 minutes during a scheduled feeding. The amount and rate are like eating a regular meal.

Continuous feedings require electronic feeding pumps (Fig. 6-7). Nasointestinal and jejunostomy tube feedings are always continuous.

Formula is given at room temperature. Cold fluids can cause cramping. Sometimes continuous feedings are kept cold with ice chips around the container. Otherwise, microbes grow in warm formula. The formula warms to room temperature as it drips from the bag and passes through the connecting tubing to the feeding tube.

Formula is added to continuous feedings every 3 to 4 hours. However, do not add new formula to formula in the bag. Otherwise, new formula is added to old formula that may be contaminated with microbes. Formula should not hang longer than 4 hours to prevent the growth of microorganisms. Some formulas have preservatives. They can hang longer. The RN tells you how long the formula can hang.

Preventing Aspiration

Aspiration is a major complication of nasogastric and nasointestinal tubes. Remember, **aspiration** is the breathing of fluid or an object into the lungs. These tubes are passed through the esophagus into the stomach or small intestine. During insertion, the tube can slip into the respiratory tract. This causes aspiration. An x-ray is the best way to determine tube placement. The x-ray is taken after the doctor or RN inserts the tube.

After insertion, the tube can move out of place from coughing, sneezing, vomiting, suctioning, and poor positioning. The tube can move from the stomach or intestines into the esophagus and then into the respiratory tract. *Therefore the RN checks tube placement before every scheduled tube feeding.* With continuous tube feedings, the RN checks tube placement every 4 to 8 hours. To check tube placement, the RN attaches a syringe to the tube and aspirates gastrointestinal secretions. Then the RN measures the pH of the secretions.

Aspiration also occurs from regurgitation. **Regurgitation** is the backward flow of food from the stomach into the mouth. This can occur with nasogastric, gastrostomy, and PEG tubes. Delayed stomach emptying and overfeeding are common causes of regurgitation. To prevent regurgitation, the person sits or is in semi-Fowler's position for the feeding. The person remains in this position for at least 1 hour after the feeding. This promotes movement of the formula through the gastrointestinal system and prevents aspiration. The left side-lying position is avoided. This position prevents the stomach from emptying.

The risk of regurgitation is less with nasointestinal and jejunostomy tubes. Formula passes directly into the small intestine. Also, formula is given at a slow rate. Remember, during digestion, food slowly passes from the stomach to the small intestine. The stomach handles larger amounts of food at one time than does the small intestine.

Observations The RN must be alert to signs and symptoms of aspiration. Other complications include diarrhea, constipation, and delayed stomach emptying. You must report the following to the RN immediately:

- Nausea
- Discomfort during the tube feeding
- Vomiting
- Diarrhea
- Distended (enlarged and swollen) abdomen
- Coughing
- Complaints of indigestion or heart burn
- Redness, swelling, drainage, odor, or pain at the ostomy site
- Elevated temperature
- Signs and symptoms of respiratory distress (see Chapter 4)
- Increased pulse rate
- Complaints of flatulence

Comfort Measures

The person with a feeding tube is usually NPO. Dry mouth, dry lips, and sore throat are sources of discomfort. Some persons are allowed hard candy or gum. The person's nursing care plan will likely include frequent oral hygiene, lubricant for the lips, and mouth rinses. The nose and nostrils also are cleaned every 4 to 8 hours as directed by the RN.

Nasogastric and nasointestinal tubes can irritate and cause pressure on the nose. Sometimes they alter the shape of the nostrils. Securing the tube helps prevent these problems. Use tape or a tube holder to secure the tube to the nose (Fig. 6-8). Tube holders have foam cushions that prevent pressure on the nose. They also eliminate the need for retaping, which irritates the nose. The tube also is secured to the person's gown. Loop a rubber band around the tube. Then pin the rubber band to the person's gown with a safety pin. Or tape the tube to the gown.

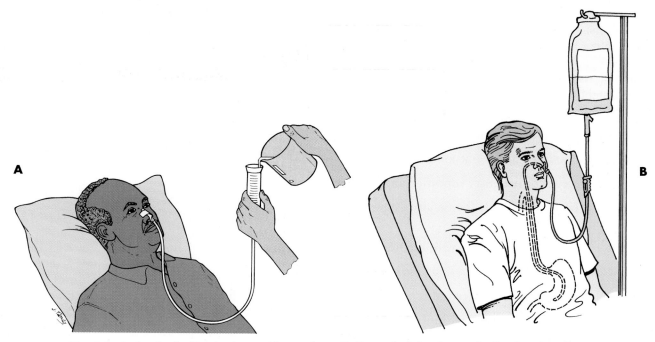

Fig. 6-6 *A, A tube feeding is given with a syringe. B, Formula drips from a feeding bag into the feeding tube.* (*B from Potter PA, Perry AG:* Fundamentals of nursing: concepts, process, and practice, *ed 4, St Louis, 1997, Mosby.*)

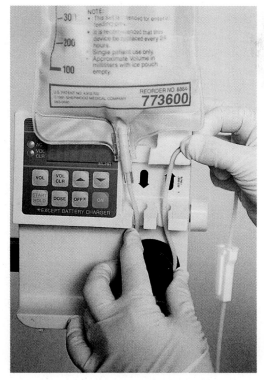

Fig. 6-7 *Feeding pump.* (*From Potter PA, Perry AG:* Fundamentals of nursing: concepts, process, and practice, *ed 4, St Louis, 1997, Mosby.*)

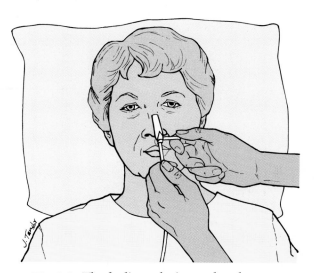

Fig. 6-8 *The feeding tube is taped to the nose.*

Giving Tube Feedings

You assist the RN with tube feedings. Some states and facilities allow assistive personnel to give tube feedings through the nasogastric and nasointestinal routes. Some also allow assistive personnel to give tube feedings through established (healed) gastrostomy and jejunostomy sites. Before you give a tube feeding:

- The procedure must be allowed by your state

- The procedure must be in your job description

- You must receive the necessary education and training

- You must be familiar with the facility's equipment and supplies

- You must review the procedure with the RN

- An RN must be available for questions and supervision

- The RN must check tube placement

The person may have intravenous infusions, drainage tubes, and a breathing tube (see Chapter 4). You must know the purpose of each tube. *Formula must enter only the feeding tube.* Otherwise the person can die. Always check and inspect the feeding tube with the RN before giving a tube feeding. Often RNs will label the person's tubes to identify their purpose. Even if tubes are labeled, you should still check and inspect the feeding tube with the RN.

focus on children Nasogastric, gastrostomy, and PEG tube feedings are more common in infants and children than are intestinal feeding tubes. Feedings are usually scheduled.

The RN tells you how to position the child. Holding the infant or small child in your lap is the preferred position. This helps comfort the child and elevates the head and chest. If the child cannot be held, the child is placed in a right side-lying position with the head and chest elevated. After the feeding, the child is positioned on the right side or in Fowler's position for 1 hour. The RN tells you how to position the child.

The RN also tells you how much formula to give. The flow rate usually is 5 ml every 5 to 10 minutes in small infants. In older infants and children, it is 10 ml per minute. Feedings take 15 to 30 minutes. A slow feeding prevents cramping, nausea, and vomiting. After the feeding, the tube is flushed with 5 to 15 ml of water.

Give infants pacifiers to suck on during the feeding. This allows the normal sucking reflex for feeding. Also, pacifiers are comforting and reduce crying.

focus on older persons The digestive process slows with aging. Stomach emptying also slows. Therefore the older person is at risk for regurgitation. Older persons may require less formula and a longer feeding time to prevent overfeeding.

focus on home care An RN is not present in the home to check tube placement. Family members are often taught to check tube placement and to give tube feedings. Follow state and agency policies for giving tube feedings in the home setting.

GIVING A TUBE FEEDING

PRE-PROCEDURE

1 Review the procedure with the RN. Ask what feeding method to use: syringe, feeding bag, or feeding pump.

2 Review the manufacturer's instructions for the feeding pump.

3 Ask the RN to verify tube placement. Check and inspect the tube with the RN to make sure you are using the right tube.

4 Explain the procedure to the person.

5 Collect the following:

- 30- or 50-ml syringe or feeding bag with tubing
- Feeding pump

- IV pole for the feeding bag
- Formula as directed by the RN
- 30 to 50 ml sterile water or other flushing solution
- Gloves (nonsterile)

6 Check the date on the formula. Do not use formula if the expiration date has passed.

7 Make sure the formula is at room temperature.

8 Clean the formula can or bottle.

9 Identify the person. Check the ID bracelet with the assignment sheet.

10 Provide for privacy.

PROCEDURE

11 Position the person in a sitting or semi-Fowler's position. The RN tells you how to position the person.

12 Put on the gloves.

13 Open the can or bottle.

14 **Give a scheduled NASOGASTRIC or GASTROSTOMY feeding using a syringe:**

  a Remove the plunger from the syringe.

  b Pinch or clamp the feeding tube. This prevents air from entering the tube and then the stomach.

  c Attach the syringe to the feeding tube.

  d Fill the syringe with formula (see Fig. 6-6, *A*).

  e Unpinch or unclamp the feeding tube.

  f Let the formula slowly pass from the syringe into the feeding tube. Raise or lower the syringe to adjust the flow rate. The higher the syringe, the faster the flow rate.

  g Add formula as necessary. Do not let the syringe empty. Otherwise air enters the feeding tube.

  h Ask the person about feelings of fullness or cramping. Pinch or clamp tubing if one or both of these occur.

  i Give formula over 20 minutes or as directed by the RN.

  j Pinch the feeding tube as the syringe empties.

  k Add the water or flushing solution to the syringe.

  l Release the feeding tube, and let the water or flushing solution clear the tube.

  m Pinch or clamp the feeding tube as the syringe empties. Do not let air enter the feeding tube.

  n Remove the syringe.

  o Cap or clamp the feeding tube.

15 **Give a scheduled NASOGASTRIC, GASTROSTOMY, or PEG feeding using a feeding bag:**

  a Close the clamp on the connecting tubing.

  b Fill the feeding bag with formula.

  c Squeeze the drip chamber so it partially fills with formula.

  d Open the clamp on the connecting tubing slowly.

  e Let formula flow through the connecting tubing to clear it of air.

  f Clamp the tubing.

  g Hang the feeding bag from the IV pole.

  h Attach the connecting tubing to the feeding tube (see Fig. 6-6, *B*).

  i Adjust the clamp on the connecting tubing to regulate the flow rate. The RN tells you the number of drops per minute. Formula is usually given over 20 minutes.

Continued

GIVING A TUBE FEEDING—CONT'D

PROCEDURE—CONT'D

j   Clamp the connecting tubing before the bag empties of formula.

k   Add water or flushing solution to the bag.

l   Unclamp the tubing, and let the water or flushing solution clear the feeding tube.

m   Clamp the connecting tubing as it empties. Do not let air enter the feeding tube.

n   Pinch or clamp the feeding tube.

o   Disconnect the connecting tube from the feeding tube.

p   Cap or clamp the feeding tube.

16 **Give a continuous NASOGASTRIC, NASOINTESTINAL, GASTROSTOMY, PEG, or JEJUNOSTOMY feeding using a pump:**

a   Follow steps 15 a through h.

b   Follow the manufacturer's instructions for threading the connecting tubing through the pump (see Fig. 6-7).

c   Set the flow rate as directed by the RN. Formula is usually given over 4 hours.

d   Add ice around the bag as directed by the RN.

e   Tell the RN when the bag is emptying. The RN assesses the person, checks for tube placement, and flushes the tube before adding more formula.

POST-PROCEDURE

17 Record the amount of formula given on the intake and output record. Also record the amount of water or flushing solution used to clear the tube.

18 Position the person as directed by the RN. The person sits or is in semi-Fowler's position. Or position the person in the right side-lying position with the head of the bed raised about 30 degrees. The position is maintained for 1 hour after the feeding.

19 Make sure the person is comfortable.

20 Place the call bell within the person's reach.

21 Make sure the bed is in its lowest position.

22 Raise or lower bed rails as instructed by the RN.

23 Unscreen the person.

24 Clean and return equipment to its proper place.

25 Remove and discard the gloves.

26 Wash your hands.

27 Report your observations to the RN.

REMOVING A NASOGASTRIC TUBE

The nasogastric tube is removed when the person can eat and swallow. The person must also be free of nausea and vomiting. The doctor gives the order to remove the tube.

Your state and job description may allow you to remove nasogastric tubes. Make sure you have the necessary training and education. Also, review the procedure with the nurse. Standard Precautions and the Bloodborne Pathogen Standard are followed.

REMOVING A NASOGASTRIC TUBE

PRE-PROCEDURE

1 Review the procedure with the RN.
2 Explain the procedure to the person.
3 Collect the following:
   - Towel
   - Tissues
   - Gloves (nonsterile)
   - Equipment for oral hygiene
4 Identify the person. Check the ID bracelet with the assignment sheet.
5 Provide for privacy.

PROCEDURE

6 Position the person in a sitting or semi-Fowler's position.
7 Put on the gloves.
8 Place the towel across the person's chest.
9 Give the person tissues so he or she can wipe the nose after the tube is removed.
10 Unpin the tube or untape the tube from the person's gown.
11 Remove tape or the tube holder from the nose.
12 Disconnect the tube if it is attached to suction.
13 Pinch the tube shut. This prevents tube contents from draining out during removal.
14 Ask the person to take a deep breath. Ask the person to hold that breath. (This closes the epiglottis, which acts like a lid over the larynx. It prevents food from entering the airway. During this procedure it prevents aspiration of stomach contents.)
15 Withdraw the tube. Use quick, smooth motions.
16 Place the tube in a biohazard bag.
17 Assist the person with oral hygiene.
18 Remove the towel.
19 Remove the gloves.

POST-PROCEDURE

20 Make sure the person is comfortable.
21 Place the call bell within reach.
22 Make sure the bed is in its lowest position.
23 Raise or lower bed rails as instructed by the RN.
24 Unscreen the person.
25 Put on clean gloves.
26 Clean and return equipment to its proper place.
27 Follow facility policy for soiled linen.
28 Remove the gloves, and wash your hands.
29 Report your observations to the RN.

SUMMARY

Enteral nutrition is ordered when the person cannot ingest normally. Formula is given through a tube into the stomach or small intestine. Assistive personnel can give tube feedings in some states and facilities.

Tube feedings are invasive procedures. They must be given through the right tube. Otherwise, the person's life is at risk. The dangers of aspiration and regurgitation also place the person's life at risk. To protect the person, you must:

- Make sure that your state allows you to perform the procedure
- Make sure that the procedure is in your job description
- Understand the procedure and what the RN expects you to do
- Review the procedure with the RN
- Ask the RN to check tube placement
- Check and inspect the tube with the RN to make sure you have the right tube

Your observations are important. The RN uses them for the nursing process. You must be alert for signs and symptoms listed on p. 110. Immediately report your observations to the RN. If problems develop during a tube feeding, stop the procedure and call for the RN. Remember, you must protect the person from harm.

REVIEW QUESTIONS

Circle the best answer.

1 You are going to give a gastrostomy tube feeding. The person is positioned in
   a Semi-Fowler's position
   b The left side-lying position
   c The right side-lying position
   d The prone position

2 What is the preferred position for giving a tube feeding to an infant or small child?
   a Elevating the head of the bed 30 degrees
   b Holding the child in your lap
   c The right side-lying position
   d Fowler's position

3 Before giving a tube feeding, you must do the following *except*
   a Review the procedure with the RN
   b Explain the procedure to the person
   c Provide for the person's privacy
   d Check tube placement

4 Formula for tube feedings is given
   a At body temperature
   b At room temperature
   c Hot
   d Cold

5 You are to give a scheduled tube feeding to an adult. How much formula is usually given during the feeding?
   a 100 ml
   b 200 ml
   c 300 ml
   d 400 ml

6 Continuous feedings are given with a
   a Syringe
   b Feeding bag
   c PEG tube
   d Feeding pump

7 Tube placement is checked to prevent
   a Aspiration
   b Regurgitation
   c Overfeeding
   d Cramping

8 To prevent regurgitation, the person is positioned
   a In semi-Fowler's position for 30 minutes after the feeding
   b In semi-Fowler's position for 1 hour after the feeding
   c In the left side-lying position for 30 minutes after the feeding
   d In the left side-lying position for 1 hour after the feeding

9 A person with a feeding tube is usually
   a Allowed a regular diet
   b On bed rest
   c NPO
   d In a coma

Circle T *if the answer is true and* F *if the answer is false.*

10 T F   Nasointestinal tube feedings are continuous.

11 T F   Jejunostomy tube feedings are scheduled.

12 T F   Jejunostomy tube feedings are given with a syringe.

13 T F   Feeding formulas provide an environment for the growth of microbes.

14 T F   Sterile technique is required when removing a nasogastric tube.

15 T F   Open formula stored in a refrigerator must be used within 24 hours.

Answers to these questions are on p. 179

7 Assisting With Intravenous Therapy

OBJECTIVES

- Know the types of IV solutions

- Know the peripheral IV sites in adults and children

- Explain the difference between peripheral IV sites and central venous sites

- Describe the equipment used in IV therapy

- Describe how you assist the RN in maintaining the IV flow rate

- Explain the safety measures necessary for IV therapy

- Identify the signs and symptoms of IV therapy complications

- Explain how to prime IV tubing

- Explain the purpose of IV dressings

- Explain how to discontinue a peripheral IV

- Perform the procedures described in this chapter

KEY TERMS

air embolism Air that enters the cardiovascular system and travels to the lungs, where it obstructs blood flow

flow rate The number of drops per minute (gtt/min)

intravenous (IV) therapy The administration of fluids into a vein; IV and IV infusion

phlebitis Inflammation *(itis)* of a vein *(phleb)*

Intravenous (IV) therapy is the administration of fluids into a vein. A needle or catheter is inserted into a vein. Fluids enter the needle or catheter and go directly into the person's circulation. *IV* and *IV infusion* also refer to IV therapy. Doctors order IV therapy to:

- Provide needed fluids when the person cannot take fluids by mouth
- Replace minerals and vitamins lost because of illness or injury
- Provide sugar for energy
- Administer medications and blood

IV therapy is given in hospital, outpatient, long-term care, and home settings. RNs are responsible for IV therapy. They start and maintain the infusion according to the doctor's orders. RNs also give IV medications and administer blood. State laws vary regarding the role of LPNs/LVNs in IV therapy. They also vary about the role of assistive personnel.

INTRAVENOUS SOLUTIONS

The doctor orders the type of IV solution to use. The solution ordered depends on the purpose of the IV therapy:

- *Nutrient solutions* are given for energy and fluid replacement. They contain carbohydrates in the form of sugar. Dextrose solutions are common.
- *Electrolyte solutions* contain minerals such as sodium, chloride, and potassium. These minerals help maintain the body's fluid balance. They are also needed for many body functions. These solutions are given when the body needs water. They also correct mineral (electrolyte) imbalances.
- *Blood volume expanders* increase the blood volume. They are used to treat hemorrhage (severe blood loss) and plasma loss. Plasma is the fluid portion of blood. Plasma loss occurs with severe burns.

Box 7-1, p. 120, lists the common IV solutions. Medications and minerals are often added to IV solutions. The pharmacist or RN adds them as ordered by the doctor. Sometimes IV solutions contain medications added by the manufacturer.

BOX 7-1 INTRAVENOUS SOLUTIONS

Nutrient solutions
- D5W—dextose 5% in water
- Dextrose 5% in 0.45% sodium chloride—5% dextrose in half-strength saline; dextrose in half-strength saline

Electrolyte solutions
- 0.9% sodium chloride—normal saline
- Lactated Ringer's
- Ringer's solution

Blood volume expanders
- Dextran
- Plasma
- Human serum albumin ❋

SITES
Peripheral IV Sites

Arm and hand veins are common IV sites for adults. The back of the hand and forearm provide useful sites (Fig. 7-1, *A*). Veins in the antecubital space (crease of the elbow) are sometimes used (Fig. 7-1, *B*). Foot veins also are sites but are avoided if possible. They are small and easily irritated by IV solutions and medications. Arm and foot sites are called *peripheral IV sites*. Periphery comes from the Greek words that mean around *(peri)* a boundary *(phery)*. The boundary is the center of the body near the heart. Therefore peripheral IV sites are located away from the center of the body.

RNs insert peripheral IVs. The site selected depends on the expected length of IV therapy, the solution, and the condition of the person's veins.

The RN tries to select a site in the person's nondominant hand or arm. Using the dominant hand interferes with some activities of daily living. In women, the arm on the side of a mastectomy (removal *[ectomy]* of a breast *[mast]*) is avoided. In persons with hemiplegia (paralysis *[plegia]* on one side of the body *[hemi]*), sites on the paralyzed side are avoided.

focus on children Scalp and dorsal foot veins (Fig. 7-2) are the peripheral sites for infants. *Dorsal* means on the back of something. Dorsal foot veins are on the back of the foot. Hand and arm veins also are used.

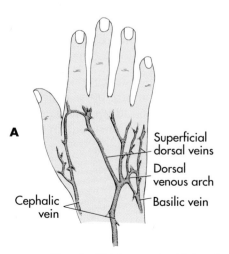

A

Superficial dorsal veins
Dorsal venous arch
Cephalic vein
Basilic vein

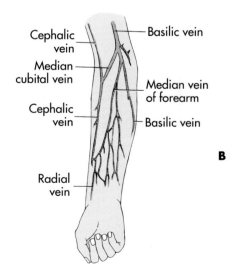

Cephalic vein
Median cubital vein
Cephalic vein
Radial vein
Basilic vein
Median vein of forearm
Basilic vein

B

Fig. 7-1 *Sites for IV therapy in adults.* **A,** *Back of the hand.* **B,** *Forearm and antecubital space.*
(*From Potter PA, Perry AG:* Fundamentals of nursing: concepts, process, and practice, *ed 4, St Louis, 1997, Mosby.*)

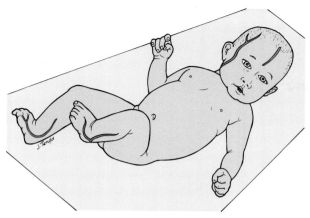

Fig. 7-2 *The scalp and foot provide IV sites in infants.*

Central Venous Sites

The subclavian vein and the internal jugular vein are *central venous sites.* These sites are close to the heart. A doctor inserts a long catheter into a central vein. The catheter tip is then threaded into the superior vena cava or right atrium (Fig. 7-3, *A* and *B*). The catheter is called a *central venous catheter* or *central line.* The cephalic and basilic veins in the arm also are used. Catheters inserted into these sites are called *peripherally inserted central catheters (PICC).* Inserted into the cephalic or basilic vein, the catheter tip is threaded into the subclavian vein or the superior vena cava (Fig. 7-3, *C*). Doctors and specially trained RNs insert PICCs.

Central venous sites are used for long-term IV therapy. They also are used to give IV medications that irritate the peripheral veins. Sometimes surgery is necessary to insert a venous catheter.

> **focus on home care** Patients can receive IV therapy in their homes. These persons often have central venous catheters. The RN teaches the patient and family about giving medications and managing the catheter.

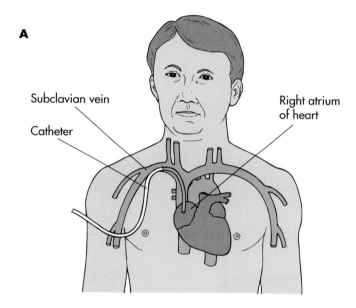

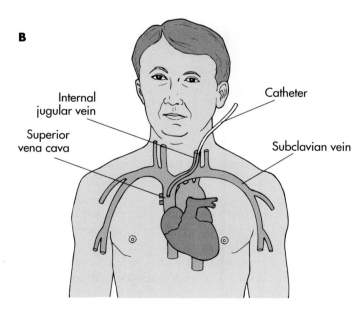

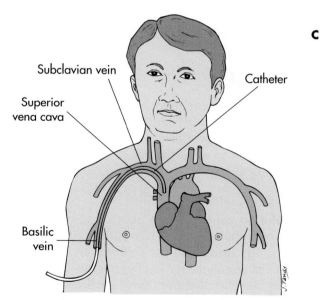

Fig. 7-3 *Central venous sites.* **A,** *Subclavian vein. The catheter tip is in the right atrium.* **B,** *Internal jugular vein. The catheter tip is in the superior vena cava.* **C,** *Basilic vein. This is a peripherally inserted central catheter (PICC).*

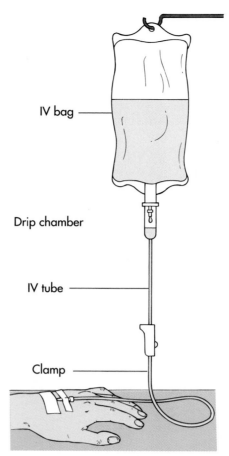

IV bag

Drip chamber

IV tube

Clamp

Fig. 7-4 *Equipment for IV therapy.*

EQUIPMENT

The basic equipment used in IV therapy includes the solution container, IV needle or catheter, infusion set (tubing), and IV pole (Fig. 7-4). Your state and facility may allow you to assist the RN in collecting and setting up equipment.

Solution Container

The solution container is a plastic bag or glass bottle. Plastic bags are common. The outside of the container is clean. The inside and the solution are sterile. Always inspect the container for contamination (Fig. 7-5). The solution must be clear and free of particles. Cloudy solutions are not used. The container's expiration date is another sign of sterility. If the expiration date has passed, the container is not used. Leaking, cracked, and open containers are not used. Return contaminated containers to the central supply area. Place a note indicating the problem on the container.

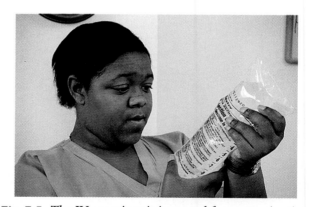

Fig. 7-5 *The IV container is inspected for contamination.*

Solution containers come in different sizes: 50, 100, 250, 500, or 1000 ml (milliliters). The size used depends on the amount of fluid ordered.

The RN tells you what type of solution to get (see Box 7-1). Doctors and RNs often use abbreviations and other

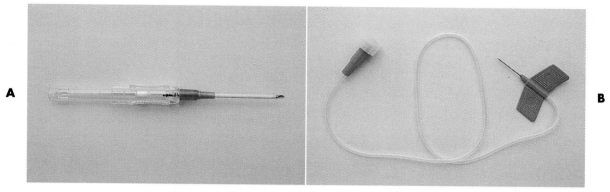

Fig. 7-6 *A*, *Intravenous catheter.* *B*, *Butterfly needle.*

names for the various IV solutions. You must clearly understand what the RN asks you to get. Always repeat the information back to the RN to make sure you understand correctly. After collecting the container, ask the RN to check the container to make sure it is the right one. If a solution contains medicine, the RN collects the container.

Catheters and Needles

A catheter or needle is inserted into a vein. An intravenous catheter is a plastic tube (Fig. 7-6, *A*). A needle fits over or is inside the catheter for insertion. After insertion, the needle is removed. Butterfly needles also are used (Fig. 7-6, *B*). However, short catheters are more common.

Catheters and needles come in different sizes. The RN selects the size based on the reasons for the IV therapy and the person's age. Smaller sizes are used for infants and children.

Infusion Sets

The infusion set (tubing) connects the solution container to the catheter or needle (see Fig. 7-4). The parts of the infusion set are shown in Figure 7-7. The *insertion spike* is sterile. A protector cap keeps the spike sterile. The cap is removed to insert the spike into the solution container.

The *needle adapter* also is sterile. A protector cap keeps it sterile. The RN removes the cap to connect the needle adapter to the intravenous catheter or needle.

Fluid drips from the solution container into the *drip chamber*. Drip chambers have macrodrips or microdrips. Depending on the manufacturer, macrodrip sets (*macro* means large) have 10 to 20 drops per milliliter (ml). Microdrip sets (*micro* means small) have 60 drops per ml. The RN uses the *clamp* to regulate the flow rate (see p. 124).

focus on children Microdrip chambers are used for infants and children.

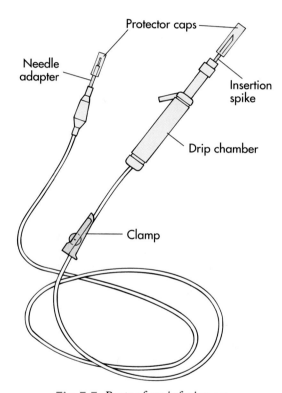

Fig. 7-7 *Parts of an infusion set.*

The IV Pole

The solution container hangs from the IV pole. *IV standard* is another name for an IV pole. IV poles are portable or part of the bed. If portable, they are kept in the supply area. An IV pole is brought to the bedside when IV therapy is started. If part of the bed, the pole is stored under the bedframe. The pole is attached to the head, foot, or side of the bed when needed.

FLOW RATE

The flow rate is measured in drops per minute. The abbreviation *gtt* means drops. It comes from the Latin word *guttae*, which means *drops*.

The doctor orders the amount of fluid to give and amount of time in which to give it. With this information, the RN decides to use a macrodrip or a microdrip chamber. The RN then calculates the flow rate. The **flow rate** is the number of drops per minute (gtt/min).

The RN sets the clamp for the flow rate. Electronic infusion devices are often used to control the flow rate (Fig. 7-8). An alarm sounds if a problem occurs with the flow rate. Tell the RN immediately if you hear the alarm. *Never change the position of the clamp or adjust any controls on infusion pumps.*

You assist the RN with IV therapy by checking the flow rate. The RN tells you the number of drops per minute. Check the flow rate by counting the number of drops in 1 full minute (Fig. 7-9). Tell the RN immediately:

- If no fluid is dripping
- If the rate is too fast
- If the rate is too slow

The person can suffer serious harm if the rate is too fast or too slow. Changes in flow rate can occur from position changes. Kinked tubes and lying on the tubing also are common problems.

ASSISTING THE RN

You assist the RN with meeting the hygiene and activity needs of persons with IVs. You may be allowed to prime IV tubing, change IV dressings, and discontinue IVs. Before you perform any of these procedures, make sure that:

- Your state allows assistive personnel to perform the procedure
- The procedure is in your job description
- You have the necessary training
- You know how to use the facility's equipment and supplies
- You review the procedure with an RN
- The RN is available to answer questions and to supervise you

You are never responsible for starting or maintaining an IV infusion. Nor do you regulate the flow rate or change IV solution containers. Assistive personnel never administer blood or IV medications. However, you assist the RN in providing safe care. The safety measures in Box 7-2 are important. Complications can occur from IV therapy. Report any of the signs and symptoms listed in Box 7-3 on p. 126 to the nurse immediately.

Remember, contact with blood is likely. Always practice Standard Precautions and follow the Bloodborne Pathogen Standard.

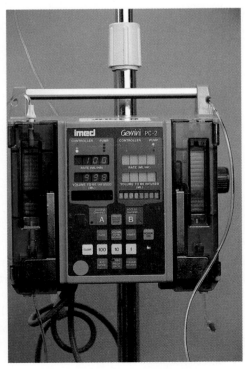

Fig. 7-8 *Electronic infusion device. (From Elkin MK, Perry AG, Potter PA: Nursing interventions and clinical skills, St Louis, 1996, Mosby.)*

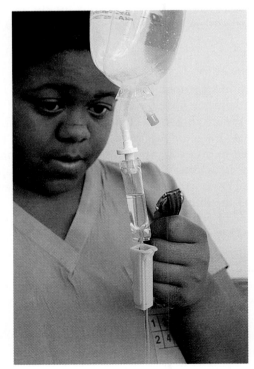

Fig. 7-9 *The flow rate is checked by counting the number of drops per minute.*

BOX 7-2 SAFETY MEASURES FOR IV THERAPY

- Always practice Standard Precautions and follow the Bloodborne Pathogen Standard.

- Do not move the needle or catheter. The position of the IV needle or catheter must be maintained when assisting a person. If the needle or catheter is moved, it may come out of the vein. Then fluid flows into the tissues (infiltration), or the flow stops.

- Follow the safety measures for restraints if a restraint is used. Sometimes the nurse splints or restrains the extremity to prevent movement of the part (Fig. 7-10). This helps prevent the needle or catheter from moving.

- Be careful not to move the needle or catheter when changing a gown.

- Protect the IV container, tubing, and needle or catheter when ambulating the person. Portable IV standards are rolled along next to the person (Fig. 7-11).

- Assist the person with turning and repositioning. The IV container is moved to the side of the bed on which the person is lying. Always allow enough slack in the tubing. The needle dislodges if pressure is exerted by the tubing.

- Notify the RN immediately if bleeding occurs from the insertion site. Be sure to follow Standard Precautions and the Bloodborne Pathogen Standard.

- Notify the RN immediately of any signs and symptoms listed in Box 7-3 on p. 126. ❋

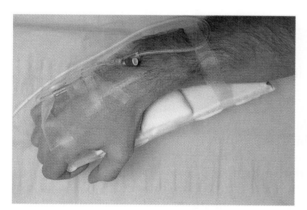

Fig. 7-10 *An armboard prevents movement at the IV site.* *(From Elkin MK, Perry AG, Potter PA:* Nursing interventions and clinical skills, *St Louis, 1996, Mosby.)*

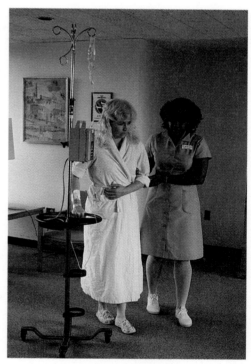

Fig. 7-11 *A person ambulating with an IV.*

BOX 7-3 SIGNS AND SYMPTOMS OF IV THERAPY COMPLICATIONS

Local—at the IV site

- Bleeding
- Puffiness or swelling
- Pale or reddened skin
- Complaints of pain at or above the IV site
- Hot or cold skin near the site

Systemic—involving the whole body

- Fever
- Itching
- Drop in blood pressure
- Tachycardia (pulse rate greater than 100 beats per minute)

- Irregular pulse
- Cyanosis
- Changes in mental function
- Loss of consciousness
- Difficulty breathing (dyspnea)
- Shortness of breath
- Decreasing or no urine output
- Chest pain
- Nausea
- Confusion ❋

Priming IV Tubing

To *prime* IV tubing means to prepare it for the administration of IV fluids. The infusion set is attached to the solution container. Fluid is allowed to flow through the tubing. This removes air from the tubing. All air is removed before the tubing is attached to the intravenous catheter or needle. Removing air includes removing bubbles. If the tubing is not primed, air enters the cardiovascular system and travels to the lungs, where it obstructs blood flow. This is called an **air embolism.** An air embolism is a life-threatening event. The person can die.

After the tubing is primed, the RN connects it to the IV catheter or needle. The RN sets the flow rate. If an infusion pump is used, the RN inserts the tubing into the pump and sets the rate.

PRE-PROCEDURE

1 Review the procedure with the RN.

2 Wash your hands.

3 Collect the following as directed by the RN:
   - IV solution (get this from the RN if it contains medications)
   - Infusion set
   - IV pole
   - Alcohol swabs
   - Disposable gloves
   - IV gown (sleeves snap close)
   - IV label

4 Check the solution container:

   a Check to see that the solution is clear and free of particles.

   b Make sure the container is unopened.

   c Make sure the container does not leak.

   d Check the container for cracks.

   e Check the expiration date.

5 Ask the RN to check the IV solution. You must make sure that you have the right solution.

6 Arrange equipment on a clean work area.

7 Identify the patient. Check the ID bracelet with the assignment sheet.

8 Explain what you are going to do.

9 Provide for privacy.

PROCEDURE

10 Help the person tend to any personal hygiene or elimination needs. Wear gloves. Clean and return equipment to its proper place. Wash your hands.

11 Help the person change into the IV gown.

12 Write the person's name and the date and time on the IV label.

13 Apply the IV label to the container. Apply it so that it can be read after hanging the container (Fig. 7-12, p. 128).

14 Open the sterile infusion set. Make sure the protective caps are on the spike and the needle adapter.

15 Open the clamp, and move it to the end of the drip chamber.

16 Close the clamp all the way.

17 Remove the protective cap from the container (Fig. 7-13, p. 128). *The opening is sterile. Do not touch the opening.*

18 Clean the rubber stopper on a glass container with an alcohol swab.

19 Remove the protective cap from the spike. *The spike is sterile. Do not touch the spike. Do not let anything touch the spike.*

20 Insert the spike into the container (Fig. 7-14, p. 128).

21 Hang the solution container on the IV pole.

22 Squeeze the drip chamber gently. Squeeze until the drip chamber is about one-half full (Fig. 7-15, p. 128).

23 Remove the protective cap from the needle adapter. Save the cap for step 28. *The adapter is sterile. Do not touch the adapter. Do not let anything touch the adapter.*

24 Hold the needle end of the tubing over a sink or container.

25 Open the clamp slowly. Open it only halfway.

26 Allow fluid to flow through the tubing until it is free of air and bubbles.

27 Close the clamp.

28 Put the protective cap on the needle adapter. *Do not touch the adapter.*

29 Check the tube for bubbles. Gently tap tubing at a bubble site to remove the bubble (Fig. 7-16, p. 128).

POST-PROCEDURE

30 Make sure the person is comfortable.

31 Make sure the call bell is within reach.

32 Raise or lower bed rails as instructed by the RN.

33 Tell the patient that the RN will start the IV.

34 Unscreen the person.

35 Tell the RN that the tubing is primed. Report any patient observations.

36 Wash your hands.

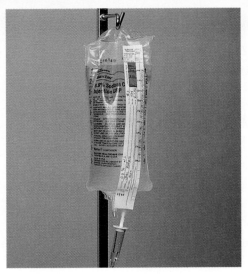

Fig. 7-12 *The IV label is applied.* (*From Potter PA, Perry AG:* Fundamentals of nursing: concepts, process, and practice, *ed 4, St Louis, 1997, Mosby.*)

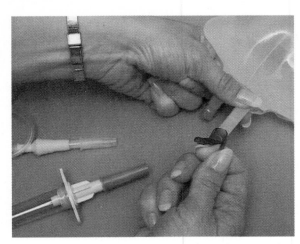

Fig. 7-13 *Removing the protective cap from the entry site of solution bag.* (*From Potter PA, Perry AG:* Fundamentals of nursing: concepts, process, and practice, *ed 4, St Louis, 1997, Mosby.*)

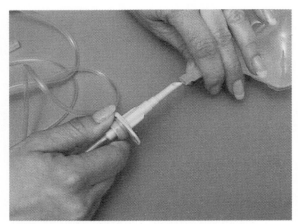

Fig. 7-14 *Inserting the spike into the entry site of the solution bag.* (*From Potter PA, Perry AG:* Fundamentals of nursing: concepts, process, and practice, *ed 4, St Louis, 1997, Mosby.*)

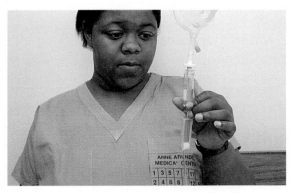

Fig. 7-15 *Squeezing the drip chamber.*

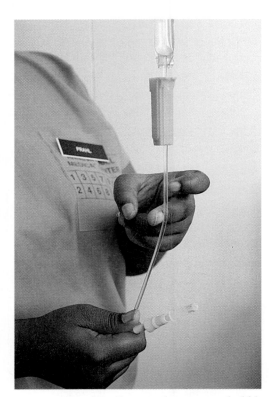

Fig. 7-16 *IV tubing is tapped to remove bubbles.*

Changing IV Dressings

After starting an IV, the RN applies a dressing to the IV site. When the IV site is changed in 2 or 3 days, the RN applies a new dressing. Sometimes IV dressings become wet, soiled, or loose. A new dressing is required. Your state and job description may allow you to change dressings at *peripheral IV sites*. The RN tells you when to change the dressing. *Do not change dressings on central venous catheters or PICCs unless allowed by your facility.*

Dressings secure the catheter or needle in place. If not secured, the catheter or needle can easily slip out of the vein. With loose dressings, the catheter or needle can move. The flow rate is affected when the catheter or needle is out of position. Also, the catheter or needle can puncture the vein. IV fluid flows into surrounding tissues. This is called *infiltration*. That is, the fluid infiltrates (goes into) other tissues. The flow rate slows. Swelling occurs at the IV site and surrounding area.

Sterile dressing changes also prevent phlebitis and infection at the venipuncture site. **Phlebitis** is an inflammation *(itis)* of the vein *(phleb)*. The person has pain, redness, and swelling at the IV site. Dressings also prevent microbes from entering the vein and bloodstream.

Gauze or transparent dressings are usually used. The IV site is easy to observe with transparent dressings. Sterile technique is used (see Chapter 2). Also see Chapter 3 for assisting with wound care. Remember to practice Standard Precautions and to follow the Bloodborne Pathogen Standard. Contact with blood is likely.

Facility procedures vary for changing IV dressings. The following procedure serves as a guideline.

focus on older persons Remember, older persons have fragile skin. Be careful when removing tape. You must prevent skin tears.

Text continued on p. 132

CHANGING A PERIPHERAL IV DRESSING

PRE-PROCEDURE

1 Review the procedure with the RN.
2 Explain the procedure to the person.
3 Wash your hands.
4 Collect the following:
   - Betadine swab (Check with the RN for patient allergies. If the person is allergic to Betadine, the RN tells you what cleaning agent to use.)
   - Alcohol swab
   - Sterile 4 × 4 or 2 × 2 gauze dressing or a transparent dressing
   - ½-inch transparent tape (if using a transparent dressing)
   - ½-inch and 1-inch nonallergic tape (if using a gauze dressing)
   - Adhesive remover
   - Cotton balls
   - Disposable gloves
   - Towel
   - Leakproof plastic bag
5 Arrange equipment on the overbed table.
6 Identify the patient. Check the ID bracelet with the assignment sheet.
7 Provide for privacy.
8 Raise the bed to a level for good body mechanics.
9 Make sure you have good lighting.

Continued

CHANGING A PERIPHERAL IV DRESSING—CONT'D

PROCEDURE

10 Cut two strips of ½-inch tape. If using a gauze dressing, also cut two strips of 1-inch tape. Hang the tape from the edge of the overbed table for later use.

11 Open the dressings and the Betadine and alcohol swabs.

12 Expose the IV site. Place the towel under the person's arm.

13 Put on the gloves.

14 Remove the soiled dressing. Be careful not to move the catheter or needle:

   a Remove the tape. Pull tape toward the IV site. Discard the tape into the plastic bag.

   b Remove the dressing. Remove one layer of gauze at a time. Touch only the outer edge of the dressing.

   c Discard the dressing into the plastic bag.

15 Observe the IV site. Check for redness, swelling, and drainage. Call for the RN to assess the site.

16 Hold the hub of the needle or catheter to keep it in place. (The hub is the plastic, colored part. See Fig. 7-6.) Use your nondominant hand. Hold the hub through step 21.

17 Remove the tape securing the catheter or needle. Discard into the plastic bag.

18 Remove any adhesive from the tape. Use cotton balls moistened with adhesive remover. Clean away from the IV site. Discard cotton balls into the plastic bag.

19 Clean the IV site with the alcohol swab. Use a circular motion starting at the IV site. Work outward about 2 inches. Let the alcohol dry. Discard used swabs into the plastic bag.

20 Clean the IV site with the Betadine swab (or other cleaning agent). Clean as in step 19. Discard used swabs into the plastic bag.

21 Let the site dry for 2 minutes.

22 Secure the catheter in place with ½-inch tape (Fig. 7-17). Your facility's procedure may omit this step for transparent dressings. If so, go to step 24:

   a Slide a tape strip—sticky side up—under the catheter hub.

   b Cross the left side of the tape over the hub to the right side.

   c Cross the right side of the tape over the hub to the left side.

   d Place a second tape strip—sticky side down—across the catheter hub.

23 Apply a gauze dressing over the catheter hub. (Do not cover the needle adapter.) Secure the dressing in place with 1-inch tape. Place the tape across the dressing.

24 Apply a transparent dressing (Fig. 7-18). Do not cover the needle adapter:

   a Apply a piece of ½-inch transparent tape across the catheter hub.

   b Apply the transparent dressing over the IV site.

   c Smooth and seal the dressing over the IV site.

25 Make a loop in the IV tubing over the dressing. Make sure the needle adapter is securely attached to the catheter hub.

26 Secure the loop to the dressing with tape. Apply the tape over the tape already on the dressing.

27 Write the date and time of the dressing change on the tape (Fig. 7-19). Also note the size of the catheter. (Get this information from the RN.)

28 Remove the towel.

29 Remove the gloves. Discard into the plastic bag.

30 Check the flow rate. Ask the RN to adjust the flow rate if needed.

POST-PROCEDURE

31 Make sure the person is comfortable.

32 Place the call bell within reach.

33 Raise or lower bed rails as instructed by the RN.

34 Lower the bed to its lowest horizontal position.

35 Unscreen the person.

36 Discard used supplies and soiled linen according to facility policy. (Wear gloves if contact with blood is likely.)

37 Wash your hands.

38 Report your observations of the IV site and old dressing to the RN. Also report any other observations or patient complaints.

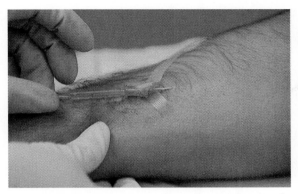

Fig. 7-17 *The catheter is secured in place with* ¹/₂*-inch tape.* *(From Elkin MK, Perry AG, Potter PA:* Nursing interventions and clinical skills, *St Louis, 1996, Mosby.)*

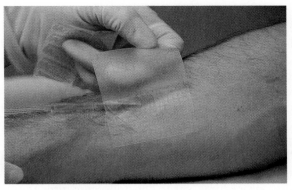

Fig. 7-18 *Transparent dressing applied over the catheter hub.* *(From Elkin MK, Perry AG, Potter PA:* Nursing interventions and clinical skills, *St Louis, 1996, Mosby.)*

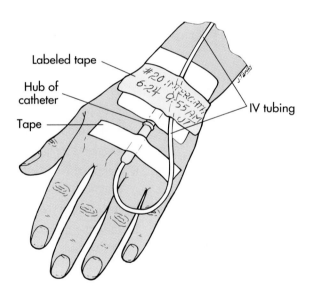

Fig. 7-19 *The dressing is labeled with date and time of the dressing change. The catheter size is also noted.*

Discontinuing Peripheral IVs

The doctor decides when to stop IV therapy. The doctor ends IV therapy when the person is no longer NPO, fluid balance is normal, or IV medications are no longer needed.

Peripheral IV sites are changed every 2 or 3 days. This reduces the risk of infection at the IV site. The RN starts the IV at a new site. The needle or catheter is removed from the old site.

The RN tells you when to discontinue an IV. The procedure should not cause the person pain or discomfort. Facility procedures vary. The following procedure is a guideline. Remember to practice Standard Precautions and follow the Bloodborne Pathogen Standard. Contact with blood is likely.

DISCONTINUING A PERIPHERAL IV

PRE-PROCEDURE

1 Review the procedure with the RN.

2 Explain the procedure to the person.

3 Wash your hands.

4 Collect the following:

- Two sterile 2 × 2 or 4 × 4 gauze dressings
- Adhesive remover
- Cotton balls
- Alcohol swabs (Check facility procedure.)
- Betadine swabs (Check with the RN for patient allergies. If the person is allergic to Betadine, the RN tells you what cleaning agent to use.)
- Tape
- Towel
- Disposable gloves
- Leakproof plastic bag

5 Arrange supplies on the overbed table.

6 Identify the patient. Check the ID bracelet with the assignment sheet.

7 Provide for privacy.

8 Raise the bed to the best level for good body mechanics.

DISCONTINUING A PERIPHERAL IV—CONT'D

PROCEDURE

9 Open the dressings, cotton balls, and alcohol and Betadine swabs.

10 Put on the gloves.

11 Expose the IV site.

12 Put the towel under the site.

13 Stop the flow of IV fluids. Close the clamp, or move it to the *OFF* position.

14 Note the amount of fluid remaining in the IV solution container.

15 Hold the hub of the catheter or needle through step 17. This prevents movement of the catheter or needle and injury to the vein.

16 Remove the tape from the dressing.

17 Remove the dressing.

18 Remove any adhesive. Use cotton balls moistened with adhesive remover. Discard cotton balls into the plastic bag.

19 Clean the IV site with an alcohol swab. Discard the swab into the plastic bag.

20 Clean the IV site with a Betadine swab. Discard the swab into the plastic bag.

21 Place a gauze square over the IV site. Hold it in place.

22 Remove the needle or catheter. Holding the hub, slowly pull the needle or catheter straight out of the vein.

23 Check the needle or catheter to make sure it is intact. This is done to make sure the needle or catheter is not left in the vein where it can travel to the lung. *Call for the RN immediately if it is not intact.*

24 Discard the catheter or needle into the sharps container in the room.

25 Apply pressure to the IV site with the gauze dressing. Apply pressure for 2 to 3 minutes. This stops bleeding from the IV site.

26 Remove the gauze dressing. Discard it into the plastic bag.

27 Apply a sterile gauze dressing to the IV site.

28 Tape the dressing in place.

29 Remove the towel.

30 Discard used supplies into the plastic bag.

31 Remove the gloves.

POST-PROCEDURE

32 Make sure the person is comfortable.

33 Place the call bell within reach.

34 Raise or lower bed rails as instructed by the RN.

35 Lower the bed to its lowest horizontal position.

36 Unscreen the person.

37 Discard used supplies, the IV solution container, and soiled linen according to facility policy. (Wear gloves for this step if contact with blood is likely.)

38 Wash your hands.

39 Report the following to the RN:

- The amount of fluid remaining in the IV bag
- Observations of the IV site
- Other observations or patient complaints

SUMMARY

IV therapy has many benefits for patients. It is often life saving. However, if not done correctly, IV therapy can seriously harm the person. Therefore IV therapy requires the knowledge and skills of RNs. Your state and facility may allow you to assist the RN with IV therapy. You are responsible for giving safe care to persons with IVs. You also observe for signs and symptoms of IV therapy complications. These are reported to the RN immediately.

Your role in assisting the RN with IV therapy may include priming IV tubes, changing peripheral IV site dressings, and discontinuing peripheral IVs. Always review these procedures with the RN before performing them. *Remember, you do not adjust the flow rate or administer IV solutions, IV medications, or blood. Nor do you discontinue IVs for persons with central venous lines.*

REVIEW QUESTIONS

Circle the best *answer.*

1 Which IV solution is given for energy and fluid replacement?
   a Electrolyte solutions
   b Normal saline solutions
   c Blood volume expanders
   d Nutrient solutions

2 The following are peripheral IV sites *except*
   a Scalp veins
   b Neck veins
   c Arm veins
   d Foot veins

3 When selecting a peripheral IV site, the RN avoids the following *except*
   a The person's dominant side
   b The person's nondominant side
   c The side of a mastectomy
   d The side of paralysis

4 You collect an IV solution container. You check the following *except*
   a For clearness and particles
   b The expiration date
   c For leaks and cracks
   d The medications added

5 Which parts of the IV infusion set are sterile?
   a The clamp and tubing
   b The clamp and spike
   c Tubing and drip chamber
   d The spike and needle adapter

6 The IV flow rate is
   a The number of gtt/ml
   b The number of gtt/min
   c The number of drops in a microdrip
   d The number of drops in a macrodrip

7 You note that the IV flow rate is too slow. You must
   a Tell the RN immediately
   b Adjust the flow rate
   c Reposition the person
   d Clamp the tubing

8 Air is removed from IV tubing to prevent
   a Phlebitis
   b An air embolism
   c PICC
   d All of the above

9 You are changing an IV dressing. Which is *false?*
   a Standard Precautions and the Bloodborne Pathogen Standard are followed.
   b A transparent dressing allows easy observation of the IV site.
   c Tape is placed over the needle adapter.
   d You check the flow rate after applying the dressing.

10 You are discontinuing an IV catheter. You remove the catheter by
   a Pulling it straight out
   b Pulling it out as you remove the dressing
   c Moving it to the left and then the right
   d Deflating the balloon

Answers to these questions are on p. 179

8 Assisting With Blood Administration

OBJECTIVES

- Define the key terms in this chapter
- Know the four blood groups in the ABO system
- Know the difference between Rh-positive and Rh-negative blood
- Know the common blood products used for transfusions
- Explain how to obtain blood from the blood bank
- Explain how to assist the RN with the administration of blood
- Identify the signs and symptoms of a transfusion reaction
- Perform the procedure described in this chapter

Key Terms

antibody A substance in the blood plasma that fights or attacks *(anti)* antigens

antigen A substance that the body reacts to

blood transfusion The intravenous administration of blood or its products

erythrocyte Red *(erythro)* blood cell *(cyte)*; carries oxygen to the cells

hemoglobin The substance in red blood cells that picks up oxygen in the lungs and carries it to the cells; it gives blood its red color

hemolysis The destruction *(lysis)* of blood *(hemo)*

leukocyte White *(leuko)* blood cell *(cyte)*; protects the body against infection

plasma The liquid portion of the blood; it carries blood cells to other body cells

platelet Thrombocyte

red blood cells (RBCs) Erythrocytes

thrombocyte A cell *(cyte)* necessary for the clotting *(thrombo)* of blood

white blood cells (WBCs) Leukocytes

The body needs adequate amounts of blood to function and survive. Blood carries nutrients, chemicals, and oxygen to the cells. Without adequate nutrition and necessary chemicals, body cells do not function properly. Cells die without oxygen. Cellular death affects organ function. The person can die.

Causes of inadequate amounts of blood are many. Blood loss often occurs from injury, disease, and surgery. When bleeding occurs, the blood normally clots to stop the bleeding. If the blood cannot clot, bleeding continues. This causes more blood loss.

As blood cells normally die off, the body must replace them. Poor nutrition affects the body's ability to produce blood cells. Also, the bone marrow must be able to produce new blood cells.

To restore normal amounts of blood and blood cells, the doctor orders the intravenous administration of blood or its products (parts). This is called a **blood transfusion.** The RN carries out the order. Blood administration is complex. The *right blood* must be given *to the right person.* Transfusion reactions are serious and life-threatening. Close observation of the person is important. So is preventing the spread of bloodborne diseases.

Your role in blood administration is to assist the RN in providing safe care to the person. You must be alert for the signs and symptoms of a transfusion reaction.

BLOOD AND BLOOD PRODUCTS

The blood consists of cells and a liquid called **plasma.** Plasma is mostly water. It carries blood cells to other body cells. Plasma also carries other substances needed by cells for proper functioning. These include nutrients (proteins, fats, and carbohydrates), hormones, and chemicals. Plasma also carries waste products to the skin and kidneys for removal from the body.

Red blood cells (RBCs) are called **erythrocytes.** Erythrocyte means red *(erythro)* cell *(cyte)*. RBCs carry oxygen to the cells. The blood gets its red color from a substance in the RBC called **hemoglobin.** As red blood cells circulate through the lungs, hemoglobin picks up oxygen. The hemoglobin carries oxygen to the cells.

The body has about 25 trillion (25,000,000,000,000) red blood cells. About $4\frac{1}{2}$ to 5 million cells are in a cubic millimeter of blood (the size of a tiny drop). These cells live for 3 to 4 months. They are destroyed by the liver and spleen as they wear out. Bone marrow produces new red blood cells. About 1 million new red blood cells are produced every second.

White blood cells (WBCs), called **leukocytes,** are colorless. Leukocyte means white *(leuko)* cell *(cyte)*. They protect the body against infection. There are 5,000 to 10,000 white blood cells in a cubic millimeter of blood. At the first sign of infection, WBCs rush to the site of the infection and multiply rapidly. The number of WBCs increases when there is an infection in the body. WBCs also are produced by the bone marrow. They live about 9 days.

Platelets (thrombocytes) are cells *(cyte)* necessary for the clotting *(thrombo)* of blood. They are also produced by the bone marrow. There are about 200,000 to 400,000 platelets in a cubic millimeter of blood. A platelet lives about 4 days.

BLOOD GROUPS AND TYPES

Blood groups and types involve the ABO system and the Rh system. These systems are important when matching blood for transfusions. If the donor blood does not match the person's blood, life-threatening reactions occur.

The ABO System

An **antigen** is a substance that the body reacts to. That is, the body attacks or fights the substance. Two types of antigens, type A and type B, are on the surface of red blood cells. If the type A antigen is in the person's blood, the person's blood group is called type A. If the type B antigen is present, the blood group is type B. Some people have both type A and type B antigens in their blood. This blood group is called type AB. The blood group type O is when neither the type A nor the type B antigens are present.

In summary, the four blood groups are:

- Type A—the type A antigen is present

- Type B—the type B antigen is present

- Type AB—the type A and the type B antigens are both present

- Type O—the type A and the type B antigens are *not* present

Antibodies are substances in the blood plasma that fight or attack *(anti)* antigens. They are normally present in the blood. Antibodies attack antigens not normally present in the person's blood. There are anti-A antibodies and anti-B antibodies:

- Blood group type A—contains anti-B antibodies

- Blood group type B—contains anti-A antibodies

- Blood group type AB—contains no antibodies

- Blood group type O—contains anti-A and anti-B antibodies

When a blood transfusion is ordered, the person must receive a compatible blood type. Otherwise, the antibodies attack the antigens. For example, a person with type A blood (type A antigens) has anti-B antibodies. If type B blood enters the person's bloodstream, the anti-B antibodies attack the type B blood. **Hemolysis** occurs. The blood *(hemo)* is destroyed *(lysis)*. This is a life-threatening reaction.

Type O blood does not contain the type A or type B antigen. Therefore it is called the *universal donor.* Persons with any blood type can receive type O blood. Even if the anti-A or anti-B antibodies are present, there are no type A or B antigens to attack in type O blood.

The Rh System

The Rh factor was first found in the rhesus (Rh) monkey. It is an antigen on the surface of red blood cells. Persons with the Rh factor are *Rh positive (Rh+)*. Persons without the Rh factor are *Rh negative (Rh−)*.

A person without the antigen (Rh negative; Rh−) must not receive blood with the antigen (Rh positive; Rh+). Otherwise, hemolysis occurs. However, a person with Rh+ blood can receive Rh− blood. This is because the antigen is not present. Antibodies have no antigen to attack.

Cross-Matching

When a person needs blood, the doctor orders laboratory *type and cross-matching* tests. Tests are done to determine the person's blood type. Then the person's blood is matched with the donor blood. This is called *cross-matching.* The tests determine if the person's blood is compatible with the donor's blood.

BLOOD PRODUCTS

The doctor orders blood or blood products (components) for the person (Fig. 8-1). The person's condition and the availability of compatible blood affect the doctor's decision. The following are often ordered:

- Whole blood

- Packed red blood cells

- Fresh frozen plasma

- Platelets

- Albumin

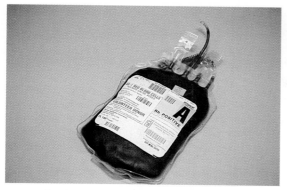

Fig. 8-1 *Blood products are packaged for administration.*

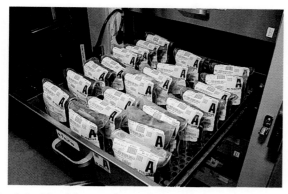

Fig. 8-2 *Blood is stored in refrigerators in the blood bank.*

ASSISTING THE RN

The RN is responsible for starting, maintaining, and ending blood transfusions. This includes assessing the person for transfusion reactions. The RN may ask you to assist in observing the person for transfusion reactions. Your state and facility may allow you to obtain blood from the blood bank.

Obtaining Blood From the Blood Bank

When type and cross-matching are complete, the laboratory notifies the RN that the blood is ready in the blood bank. The blood bank is located in the laboratory (Fig. 8-2). Remember, *the right blood must be given to the right person.* You must obtain the right blood from the blood bank. Strict identification measures are practiced.

Time is critical when a person needs blood. You must go straight to the blood bank and immediately report back to the RN. Do not stop on the way to and from the blood bank. Do not stop to visit, do other errands, use the restroom, have a break, or any other activity. Minutes count.

OBTAINING BLOOD FROM THE BLOOD BANK

PROCEDURE

1 Review the procedure with the RN.
2 Take the blood requisition form to the blood bank.
3 Tell the following to the laboratory technician:
   • Who you are
   • What you want
   • That you have a requisition for blood or a blood product
4 Check the requisition form and the blood bag label with the laboratory technician (Fig. 8-3). Follow facility policy. Read the following out loud:
   a The person's name—last name, first name, and middle initial
   b The person's identification number
   c The person's blood type—A, B, AB, or O
   d The person's Rh factor—Rh+ or Rh−
   e The blood donor number
   f Expiration date on the blood
5 Thank the technician for helping you.
6 Return immediately to the nursing unit.
7 Give the blood to the RN.
8 Wash your hands.

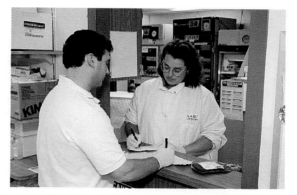

Fig. 8-3 *Blood is checked with the laboratory technician.*

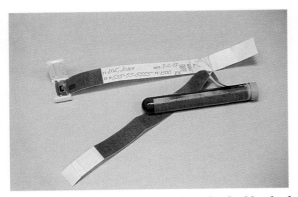

Fig. 8-4 *The patient is given an ID bracelet for blood administration when the blood specimen is drawn for type and cross-matching. All blood products for the patient have a number that matches the ID bracelet.*

Transfusion Reactions

Transfusion reactions occur when the person's blood is not compatible with donor blood. Antibodies in the person's blood attack and destroy antigens in the donor blood. Blood cells are destroyed in the process (hemolysis). The person's life is seriously threatened. Death can occur.

Giving the wrong blood to the wrong person is a common cause of transfusion reactions. To prevent this, the blood bag tag is again checked with the blood requisition form before the blood is administered. Identifying information is also checked with the person's ID bracelet (Fig. 8-4). This is usually done by two RNs at the person's bedside. Facility policy may allow you to check the blood with the RN. You must be very careful. If the information does not match exactly, tell the RN.

Before starting the transfusion, the person's vital signs are measured. The RN may ask you to do this. These vital signs serve as a baseline. The RN compares vital signs taken during the transfusion with the baseline vital signs. A change in any vital sign signals a transfusion reaction.

The first 15 minutes of the transfusion is the most critical time for the person. The RN carefully assesses the person for signs and symptoms of a transfusion reaction. The person's vital signs are measured often.

Vital signs are measured during the transfusion and for 1 hour after the transfusion. It usually takes about 2 hours to transfuse 1 unit (1 bag) of blood. The RN may ask you to assist with measuring vital signs. The RN tells you how often to measure them—usually every 15 or 30 minutes. These vital signs are recorded on a flow sheet. You must measure vital signs on time and accurately.

BOX 8-1 SIGNS AND SYMPTOMS OF TRANSFUSION REACTIONS

- Chills
- Fever
- Headache
- Back pain or backache
- Chest pain
- Dyspnea (difficulty breathing)
- Tachypnea (rapid breathing)
- Coughing
- Tachycardia (rapid pulse)
- Hypotension (low blood pressure)
- Loss of consciousness
- Cardiac arrest
- Flushing
- Blood in the urine
- Itching
- Hives (urticaria)
- Wheezing
- Warm, flushed skin
- Anxiety
- Muscle pain
- Nausea
- Vomiting
- Abdominal cramping
- Diarrhea ✳

When you measure vital signs, also check the flow rate (see Chapter 7). The RN tells you the number of drops per minute. Immediately tell the RN if:

- The flow rate is too fast
- The flow rate is too slow
- The transfusion has stopped
- The bag is close to empty

You also must be alert for signs and symptoms of transfusion reactions (Box 8-1). Report any sign or symptom immediately to the RN. The RN will stop the transfusion.

SUMMARY

Blood transfusions can save a person's life. They can also kill if the wrong blood is given to the wrong person. Therefore blood administration requires the knowledge, skills, and judgment of RNs. Your state and job description may allow you to assist the RN.

You must follow the RN's directions carefully and exactly. Always be alert for signs and symptoms of a transfusion reaction. Report any sign or symptom immediately to the RN.

REVIEW QUESTIONS

Circle the best *answer.*

1 Which carry oxygen to the cells?
  a Antibodies
  b Antigens
  c Hemoglobin
  d Platelets

2 The liquid portion of blood is called
  a Plasma
  b Erythrocytes
  c Hemoglobin
  d Hemolysis

3 Which is necessary for blood clotting?
  a Plasma
  b Erythroctyes
  c Hemoglobin
  d Platelets

4 A person's blood has the type B antigen. The person's blood type is
  a Type A
  b Type B
  c Type AB
  d Type O

5 A person with type O blood
  a Has the type A and type B antigens
  b Is Rh+
  c Has no antigens
  d Is Rh−

6 Who can receive type O blood?
  a Persons with type A blood or type B blood
  b Persons with type AB blood

  c Persons with type O blood
  d All of the above

7 You are asked to obtain blood from the blood bank. The following are checked with the laboratory technician *except*
  a The person's blood type
  b The person's Rh factor
  c The person's ID bracelet
  d The blood's expiration date

8 The most critical time for a transfusion reaction is
  a The first 15 minutes of the infusion
  b The first hour of the infusion
  c The last hour of the infusion
  d The first hour after the infusion

9 A patient is receiving a blood transfusion. The person complains of a backache and chills. What should you do?
  a Measure the person's vital signs.
  b Tell the RN immediately.
  c Stop the transfusion.
  d Ask about other signs and symptoms.

10 The following are signs and symptoms of a transfusion reaction *except*
  a Wound drainage
  b Hypotension
  c Tachycardia
  d Chest pain

Answers to these questions are on p. 179

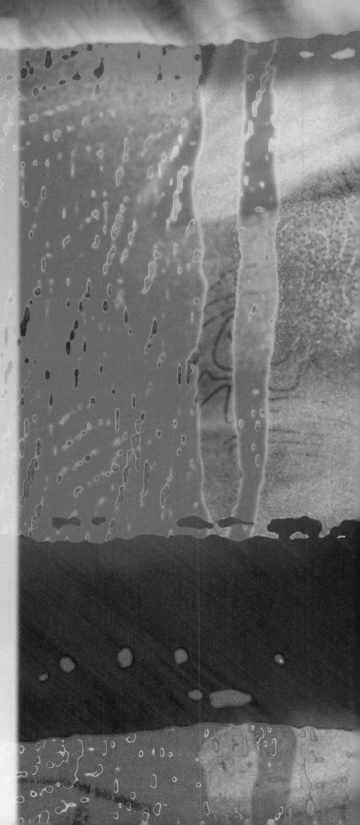

9 Collecting and Testing Blood Specimens

OBJECTIVES

- Define the key terms in this chapter
- Identify the sources of blood specimens
- Identify the sites for a skin puncture
- Describe three venipuncture methods
- Explain how to collect tubes for blood specimens
- Identify the information required for labeling blood specimens
- Identify the common venipuncture sites for collecting blood specimens
- Explain how to select a venipuncture site
- Explain the importance of blood glucose testing
- Describe two methods of blood glucose testing
- Explain the rules for blood glucose testing
- Perform the procedures described in this chapter

KEY TERMS

callus A thick, hardened area on the skin

hematology The study *(ology)* of blood *(hemat)*

hematoma A swelling *(oma)* that contains blood *(hemat)*

lancet A short, disposable blade

palpate To feel or touch using your hands or fingers

tourniquet A constricting device applied to a limb to control bleeding

venipuncture A technique in which a vein *(veni)* is punctured

Hematology is the study of *(ology)* blood *(hemat)*. Blood tests are very common in health care. They play a role in preventing disease and in detecting and treating disease. Blood tests are ordered by doctors. Most tests are done in the laboratory. Some are done at the bedside or in home settings by nurses and assistive personnel.

Blood specimens are drawn by laboratory personnel and nurses. Many states and facilities allow assistive personnel to obtain blood specimens. Before collecting and testing blood specimens, make sure:

- Your state allows assistive personnel to perform the procedures
- The procedures are in your job description
- You have the necessary training
- You know how to use the facility's equipment
- You review the procedures with an RN
- The RN is available to answer questions and to supervise you

Standard Precautions and the Bloodborne Pathogen Standard are followed when collecting and testing blood specimens. Contact with blood is likely.

SOURCES OF BLOOD SPECIMENS

Most blood tests require blood obtained from skin punctures or venipunctures. Sometimes arterial blood is needed. Persons with respiratory diseases and those on mechanical ventilation often require blood gas analysis. The tests measure the amount of oxygen and carbon dioxide in the arterial blood. The specimen is collected by making an arterial stick. Laboratory technicians, RNs, and respiratory therapists with special training do arterial sticks.

Skin Punctures

With skin punctures, a few drops of capillary blood are obtained. A fingertip is the most common site for skin punctures. The earlobe also is a site. These sites provide easy access and do not require clothing removal. The patient feels a sharp pinch. Discomfort is brief.

Inspect the site carefully. Look for signs of trauma. Avoid sites that are swollen, bruised, cyanotic (bluish color), scarred, or calloused. Blood flow to these areas is poor. A **callus** is a thick, hardened area on the skin. Calluses often form over areas that are used frequently, such as the tips of the thumbs and index fingers. Therefore the thumbs and index fingers are not good sites for skin punctures. Also avoid sites that have skin breaks.

Avoid using the center, fleshy part of the fingertip. The site has many nerve endings. A puncture at the site is painful. Use the side or top of the fingertip (Fig. 9-1).

A sterile lancet is used to puncture the skin (Fig. 9-2). A **lancet** is a short, pointed blade. Because the blade is short, it punctures but does not cut the skin. The lancet is enclosed in a protective cover. You do not touch the actual blade. Different types of lancets are available. All are disposable. A lancet is used once and discarded into the sharps container.

focus on children The heel is used for skin punctures in infants. Finger and earlobe sites are used for children. Give the child a choice of sites. Then let the child choose the site for the skin puncture. This gives the child a sense of control.

focus on older persons Older persons often have poor circulation in their fingers. Applying a warm wash cloth or washing the hands in warm water helps increase blood flow.

focus on home care An RN teaches patients and family members to do skin punctures in the home setting.

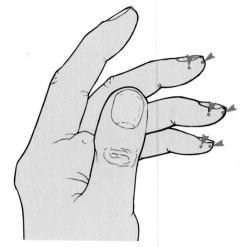

Fig. 9-1 *Sites for skin punctures.*

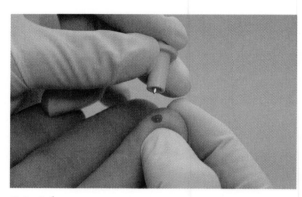

Fig. 9-2 *A lancet. (From Zakus SM:* Clinical procedures for medical assistants, *ed 3, St Louis, 1995, Mosby.)*

PERFORMING A SKIN PUNCTURE

PRE-PROCEDURE

1 Review the procedure with the RN.
2 Explain the procedure to the person.
3 Wash your hands.
4 Collect the following:
   - Sterile lancet
   - Alcohol wipes
   - Disposable gloves
   - Cotton balls
   - Washcloth
   - Soap, towel, and wash basin
5 Read the manufacturer's instructions for the lancet.
6 Arrange supplies in a convenient location.
7 Identify the person. Check the ID bracelet with the assignment sheet or laboratory requisition form.
8 Provide for privacy.

PROCEDURE

9 Help the person assume a comfortable position.

10 Ask the person to wash his or her hands. Provide necessary supplies and equipment.

11 Open the lancet and alcohol wipes.

12 Put on the gloves.

13 Inspect the person's fingers. Select a skin puncture site.

14 Warm the finger or earlobe if it is cold. To warm the part, gently rub it or apply a warm washcloth.

15 Massage the hand and finger toward the puncture site. This brings more blood to the site.

16 Lower the finger so the hand is below the person's waist. This increases blood flow to the site.

17 Hold the finger with your thumb and forefinger (see Fig. 9-2). Use your nondominant hand. Hold the finger until step 23.

18 Clean the site with alcohol. *Do not touch the site after cleaning.*

19 Allow the site to dry.

20 Pick up the sterile lancet.

21 Place the lancet against the side of the finger or the top of the finger tip (Fig. 9-3).

22 Puncture the skin by pushing the button on the lancet. (Follow the manufacturer's instructions.)

23 Wipe away the first blood drop. Use a cotton ball.

24 Apply gentle pressure below the puncture site.

25 Allow a large drop of blood to form (Fig. 9-4).

26 Collect and test the specimen (see p. 154).

27 Apply pressure to the puncture site until bleeding stops. Use a cotton ball. If the person is able, let the person continue to apply pressure to the site.

28 Discard the lancet into the sharps container.

29 Discard the cotton balls following facility policy. Remember, they contain blood.

30 Remove and discard the gloves.

POST-PROCEDURE

31 Help the person to a comfortable position.

32 Make sure the call bell is within reach.

33 Raise or lower bed rails as instructed by the RN.

34 Lower the bed to its lowest horizontal position.

35 Unscreen the person.

36 Discard used supplies. Clean and return the bath basin to its proper place.

37 Follow facility policy for soiled linen.

38 Wash your hands.

39 Report the following to the RN:

- The time the specimen was collected
- The test results (see p. 154).
- The site used
- How the person tolerated the procedure
- Other observations or patient complaints

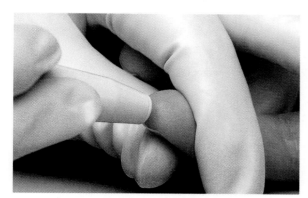

Fig. 9-3 *Puncturing the skin with a lancet. (From Elkin MK, Perry AG, Potter PA:* Nursing interventions and clinical skills, *St Louis, 1996, Mosby.)*

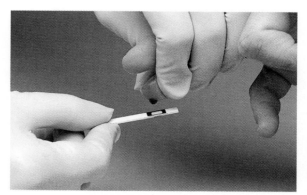

Fig. 9-4 *A large drop of blood forms. (From Elkin MK, Perry AG, Potter PA:* Nursing interventions and clinical skills, *St Louis, 1996, Mosby.)*

Venipunctures

Venipunctures are done when large amounts of blood are needed. **Venipuncture** is a technique in which a vein *(veni)* is punctured with a needle.

The needle is attached to a syringe or a Vacutainer. With the syringe method, you pull back on the plunger to withdraw blood into the barrel (Fig. 9-5). (Review parts of a syringe on p. 99.) After the blood is collected, it is transferred to a test tube.

With a Vacutainer, blood flows into the tube (Fig. 9-6). The Vacutainer system has a needle, needle and tube holder, and evacuated tube with rubber stopper (Fig. 9-7). In evacuated tubes, air is removed, creating a vacuum. When a vein is punctured, blood flows into the tube. The Vacutainer system allows the collection of many blood specimens with one venipuncture. After a tube fills, it is removed and a new one attached to the holder.

Selecting collection tubes Blood collection tubes come in different sizes. The blood test ordered determines the amount of blood needed. Also, some tests require additives. Additives are chemicals that are added to the collection tube. The chemicals preserve the blood until testing.

In the Vacutainer system, the tubes contain the necessary additives. The rubber stoppers are color-coded. Red, lavender, blue, green, gray, and yellow are common colors. The color-coding signals the type of additive, the amount of blood to collect, and the recommended blood tests. Color-coding may vary with facilities. Always follow your facility's procedures. Check the Vacutainer tube guide (Fig. 9-8) when selecting tubes for blood tests.

After selecting the collection tubes, place them in order of use. The order is important to prevent tube contamination. Different tubes have different additives. The additives must not be transferred from one tube to another. Follow facility procedures for the order in which to collect blood specimens.

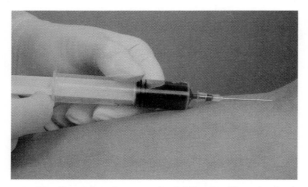

Fig. 9-5 *Needle and syringe method. Blood collects in the barrel as the plunger is pulled back. (From Zakus SM:* Clinical procedures for medical assistants, *ed 3, St Louis, 1995, Mosby.)*

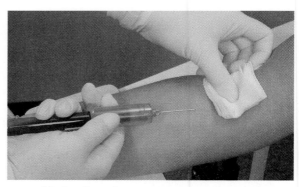

Fig. 9-6 *Blood collects in a Vacutainer tube. (From Zakus SM:* Clinical procedures for medical assistants, *ed 3, St Louis, 1995, Mosby.)*

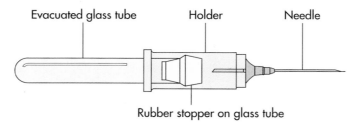

Evacuated glass tube   Holder   Needle

Rubber stopper on glass tube

Fig. 9-7 *Parts of the Vacutainer. (From Zakus SM:* Clinical procedures for medical assistants, *ed 3, St Louis, 1995, Mosby.)*

Labeling collection tubes Before blood specimens are sent to the laboratory, the collection tube must be labeled with the person's identifying information. Labeling is done at the bedside after the specimens are collected. Labeling is necessary to make sure that the right tests are done for the right person. Otherwise, wrong test results are reported for the person. This leads to the wrong treatment. The person can suffer serious harm.

Follow your facility's procedure for labeling blood specimens. Labeling includes:

- The person's full name—last name, first name, and middle name or initial

- The person's ID number

- The person's bed and room number

- The person's age

- The person's gender (male or female)

- Doctor's name

- Date and time the specimen was collected

- Your name or initials

- Blood test ordered

Selecting a venipuncture site The basilic and cephalic veins in the antecubital space are the most common venipuncture sites (Fig. 9-9). These veins are large and near the skin surface. Hand veins offer alternative sites.

Before selecting a vein, select the arm that you will use. Avoid the arm on the side of a mastectomy (removal of a breast) or on the side of hemiplegia. If a person has an IV infusion, do not use that arm. Do not use the arm with an access site for hemodialysis. Always discuss site selection with the RN. The RN tells you what side to avoid.

Inspect the arm you will use. Look for skin breaks and hematomas. A **hematoma** is a swelling (*oma*) that contains blood (*hemat*). Do not use sites with skin breaks or hematomas.

To select a vein, apply a tourniquet (Fig. 9-10). A **tourniquet** is a constricting device applied to a limb to control bleeding. The device is applied above the bleeding site. It prevents arterial blood flow to the part below the tourniquet. Likewise, it prevents venous blood from returning to the heart. Therefore tourniquets are useful for venipunctures. The veins fill with blood and distend (enlarge). They are firmer and easier to see and feel. The tourniquet is removed after collecting the blood specimen.

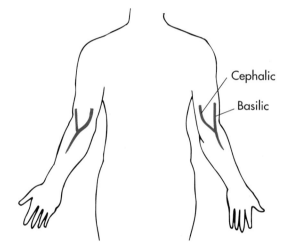

Fig. 9-9 *Veins in the antecubital space.* (*From Cooper MG, Cooper DE, Burrows NJ:* The medical assistant, *ed 6, St Louis, 1993, Mosby.*)

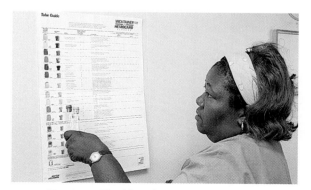

Fig. 9-8 *Checking the Vacutainer guide.*

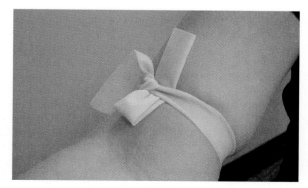

Fig. 9-10 *A tourniquet is applied to select a venipuncture site.* (*From Zakus SM:* Clinical procedures for medical assistants, *ed 3, St Louis, 1995, Mosby.*)

When used for venipunctures, tourniquets serve to prevent venous blood flow—not arterial blood flow. The tourniquet must be tight so that the veins distend. However, you should feel the radial pulse. If you do not feel a radial pulse, the arm is not getting arterial blood. Release and reapply the tourniquet. Feel for the radial pulse again. A tourniquet is applied no longer than 1 minute.

To select a vein in the antecubital space, apply a tourniquet 3 to 4 inches above the elbow. Then ask the person to open and close a fist. With the fist closed, look and feel for a vein. Look for a straight vein. The vein should feel full and firm. It should be elastic and rebound (spring back) after you palpate it. To **palpate** means to feel or touch using your hands or fingers. You use your fingers to palpate veins (Fig. 9-11). Avoid veins that are:

- Small and narrow—they are usually fragile

- Weak—weak veins are soft and do not rebound

- Sclerosed—*sclero* means hardened; sclerosed veins are hard and rigid

- Easy to roll—the vein rolls when palpated

focus on children Children are often afraid of needles. Explain what you are going to do. Ask a parent or another staff member to hold and comfort the child. Use toys or books to distract the child. Also keep the needle out of the child's sight for as long as possible. Perform the venipuncture and collect the blood quickly.

Children fear the loss of blood. Explain that they have a lot of blood and that their bodies constantly make blood. Placing an adhesive bandage over the site is comforting. It reassures the child that blood will not leak from the body.

focus on older persons Older persons often have fragile or sclerosed veins. Ask the RN to assist you with site selection.

Text continued on p.154

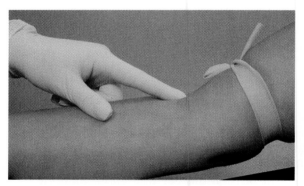

Fig. 9-11 *Palpating a vein. (From Zakus SM:* Clinical procedures for medical assistants, *ed 3, St Louis, 1995, Mosby.)*

COLLECTING BLOOD SPECIMENS WITH A NEEDLE AND SYRINGE

PRE-PROCEDURE

1 Review the procedure with the RN. Discuss site selection.

2 Explain the procedure to the person.

3 Wash your hands.

4 Collect the following:

- Alcohol swabs
- Tourniquet
- Sterile 2 × 2 gauze dressings
- Tape or adhesive bandage
- Sterile needle
- Sterile syringe
- Color-coded vacuum test tube (check the expiration date)
- Laboratory requisition forms
- Labels for the blood specimens
- Towel
- Disposable gloves
- Leakproof plastic bag
- Portable sharps container (optional)

5 Complete the labels for the blood specimens.

6 Arrange equipment on the overbed table. If using a blood collection tray, place it on the bedside table or the chair. (The tray is used for many patients. It can contaminate the overbed table that is used for eating and other nursing procedures.)

7 Identify the person. Check the ID bracelet with the laboratory requisition forms.

8 Provide for privacy.

9 Raise the bed to the best level for good body mechanics.

PROCEDURE

10 Help the person assume a comfortable procedure. The person should be supine, sitting, or in semi-Fowler's position.

11 Inspect both arms for skin breaks and hematomas. Ask the person if he or she prefers the right or left arm for the venipuncture.

12 Choose the side you will use. Position the overbed table so you can reach supplies easily.

13 Place a rolled towel under the arm.

14 Position the arm. Extend the arm with the palm side up.

15 Prepare the supplies:

a Open the alcohol swabs.

b Open the sterile gauze squares.

c Open the adhesive bandage.

d Open the needle and syringe package.

e Attach the needle to the syringe.

16 Put on the gloves.

17 Apply the tourniquet 3 or 4 inches above the elbow:

a Cross one end tightly over the other.

b Tuck the upper end under the band to form a half bow (see Fig. 9-10).

18 Palpate the radial pulse. Release and reapply the tourniquet if you do not feel a pulse.

19 Ask the person to open and close the fist a few times.

20 Look and palpate for a vein in the antecubital space (see Fig. 9-11).

21 Select a vein. Avoid veins that are narrow, weak, sclerosed, or rolling.

22 Release the tourniquet if it has been on longer than 1 minute.

23 Wait 1 minute before reapplying the tourniquet.

24 Reapply the tourniquet.

25 Palpate the vein again.

26 Clean the site with an alcohol swab. Clean in a circular motion from the site outward about 2 inches. *Do not touch the site after cleaning.*

27 Let the site dry.

28 Pick up the needle and attached syringe.

29 Remove the needle cover. Pull it straight off. *Do not touch the needle.*

30 Pull the skin over the site taut. Use the thumb or first two fingers of your nondominant hand (Fig. 9-12, p. 151). Hold the site taut until step 33.

Continued

COLLECTING BLOOD SPECIMENS WITH A NEEDLE AND SYRINGE—CONT'D

PROCEDURE—CONT'D

31 Hold the needle and syringe so that the needle bevel is up. (The bevel is the pointed end.)

32 Position the needle at a 15- to 30-degree angle to the person's arm.

33 Insert the needle into the vein gently and smoothly (Fig. 9-13).

34 Pull back on the plunger slowly to withdraw blood (Fig. 9-14). Use your nondominant hand.

35 Release the tourniquet. Pull on the half bow.

36 Continue to pull back on the plunger until you have withdrawn the necessary amount of blood. Keep the needle stable so it does not move.

37 Hold a gauze square over the puncture site. Do not apply pressure.

38 Pull the needle straight out.

39 Apply pressure to the venipuncture site with the gauze square. Ask the person to apply pressure to the arm. Bleeding stops in 1 to 3 minutes.

40 Transfer blood from the syringe into the vacuum tube. Be very careful not to stick yourself with the needle. Follow facility policy for tube order (see p. 146).

   a Method 1:

     1) Insert the needle through the rubber stopper on the tube.

     2) Let the vacuum tube fill (Fig. 9-15, p. 146).

     3) Discard the needle and syringe into the sharps container. *Do not recap the needle.*

   b Method 2:

     1) Remove the needle from the syringe. Discard it into the sharps container. *Do not recap the needle.*

     2) Remove the rubber stopper from the tube.

     3) Inject blood directly into the tube by pushing down on the plunger.

     4) Insert the rubber stopper.

     5) Check the outside of the tube for blood. Remove any blood with alcohol swabs.

41 Identify the tubes with additives. Mix the blood and additives by gently inverting each tube back and forth. Follow the manufacturer's instructions for the number of times to invert the tube (usually 8 to 10 times). Do not shake the tube.

42 Check the venipuncture site for bleeding.

43 Remove the gauze square.

44 Apply a new gauze square or adhesive bandage. Secure the gauze square with tape.

45 Discard the syringe into the sharps container if you have not yet done so.

46 Apply labels to the blood specimens.

47 Put the specimens into the plastic bag (if this is your facility's policy).

48 Remove the towel under the person's arm. Follow facility policy for soiled linen. The towel may contain blood.

49 Discard cotton balls, gauze, and alcohol swabs following facility policy. These supplies may contain blood.

50 Remove and discard the gloves.

COLLECTING BLOOD SPECIMENS WITH A NEEDLE AND SYRINGE—CONT'D

POST-PROCEDURE

51 Assist the person to a comfortable position.

52 Place the call bell within reach.

53 Raise or lower bed rails as instructed by the RN.

54 Lower the bed to its lowest horizontal position.

55 Discard any other used supplies.

56 Unscreen the person.

57 Take the blood specimens to the nurses' station.

58 Report the following to the RN:

- The time the specimens were collected

- The site used

- The amount of bleeding at the site

- Any signs of hematoma

- How the person tolerated the procedure

- Patient complaints of pain at the site

- Any other observations or patient complaints

- What you did with the specimens

59 Take or send the specimens to the laboratory as directed by the RN.

60 Wash your hands.

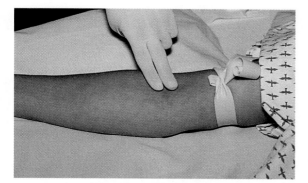

Fig. 9-12 *Pulling the skin taut over the venipuncture site.* (*From Perry AG, Potter PA:* Clinical nursing skills and techniques, *ed 4, St Louis, 1996, Mosby.*)

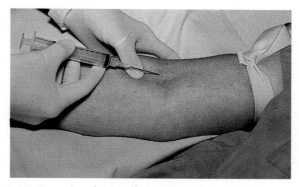

Fig. 9-13 *Inserting the needle into the vein.* (*From Perry AG, Potter PA:* Clinical nursing skills and techniques, *ed 4, St Louis, 1996, Mosby.*)

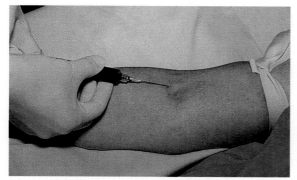

Fig. 9-14 *Pulling back on the plunger to withdraw blood.* (*From Perry AG, Potter PA:* Clinical nursing skills and techniques, *ed 4, St Louis, 1996, Mosby.*)

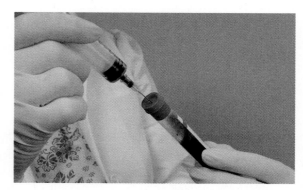

Fig. 9-15 *Transferring blood from the syringe into the vacuum tube.* (*From Zakus SM:* Clinical procedures for medical assistants, *ed 3, St Louis, 1995, Mosby.*)

COLLECTING BLOOD SPECIMENS USING THE VACUTAINER SYSTEM

PRE-PROCEDURE

1 Review the procedure with the RN. Discuss site selection.

2 Explain the procedure to the person.

3 Wash your hands.

4 Collect the following:
   - Alcohol swabs
   - Tourniquet
   - Sterile 2 × 2 gauze dressings
   - Tape or adhesive bandage
   - Vacutainer tube holder
   - Sterile double-ended Vacutainer needle
   - Vacutainer tubes (check the expiration date)
   - Laboratory requisition forms
   - Labels for the blood specimens
   - Towel
   - Disposable gloves
   - Leakproof plastic bag

5 Complete the labels for the blood specimens.

6 Arrange equipment on the overbed table.

7 Identify the person. Check the ID bracelet with the laboratory requisition forms.

8 Provide for privacy.

9 Raise the bed to the best level for good body mechanics.

PROCEDURE

10 Follow steps 10 through 14 in *Collecting Blood Specimens With a Needle and Syringe.*

11 Prepare the supplies:
   a Open the alcohol swabs.
   b Open the sterile gauze squares.
   c Open the adhesive bandage.
   d Open the double-ended needle.
   e Attach the needle to the Vacutainer tube holder (Fig. 9-16).
   f Place the first tube to be used inside the holder. Do not attach it to the needle.
   g Arrange tubes in order of use. Follow facility policy.

12 Follow steps 16 through 27 in *Collecting Blood Specimens With a Needle and Syringe.*

13 Pick up the Vacutainer needle and tube holder.

14 Remove the needle cover. Pull it straight off. *Do not touch the needle.*

15 Pull the skin over the site taut. Use the thumb or forefinger of your nondominant hand. Hold the site taut until step 19.

16 Hold the needle so that the needle bevel is up. (The bevel is the pointed end.)

17 Position the needle at a 15- to 30-degree angle to the person's arm.

18 Insert the needle into the vein gently and slowly (Fig. 9-17).

19 Push the tube forward onto the end of the needle in the holder. Push gently.

20 Let the tube fill with blood (Fig. 9-18).

21 Remove the filled tube from the holder. Grasp it firmly.

22 Insert the next tube. Repeat steps 19 through 22 for the other tubes.

23 Release the tourniquet after the last tube fills.

24 Hold a gauze square over the puncture site. Do not apply pressure.

25 Pull the needle straight out.

26 Apply pressure to the venipuncture site with the gauze square. Ask the person to apply pressure to the arm. Bleeding stops in 1 to 3 minutes.

27 Remove the last tube from the tube holder. *Do not recap the needle.*

28 Discard the needle and tube holder into the sharps container.

29 Identify the tubes with additives. Mix the blood and additives by gently inverting each tube back and forth. Follow the manufacturer's instructions for the number of times to invert the tube (usually 8 to 10 times). Do not shake the tube.

COLLECTING BLOOD SPECIMENS USING THE VACUTAINER SYSTEM—CONT'D

PROCEDURE—CONT'D

30 Check the venipuncture site for bleeding.

31 Remove the gauze square.

32 Apply a new gauze square or adhesive bandage. Secure the gauze square with tape.

33 Apply labels to the blood specimens.

34 Put the specimens into the plastic bag (if this is your facility's policy).

35 Remove the towel under the person's arm. Follow facility policy for soiled linen. The towel may contain blood.

36 Discard cotton balls, gauze, and alcohol swabs following facility policy. These supplies may contain blood.

37 Remove and discard the gloves.

POST-PROCEDURE

38 Follow steps 51 through 60 in *Collecting Blood Specimens With a Needle and Syringe.*

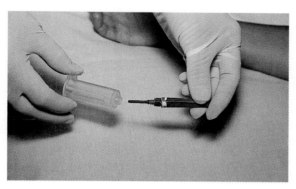

Fig. 9-16 *Attaching the double-ended needle to the Vacutainer tube holder. (From Perry AG, Potter PA:* Clinical nursing skills and techniques, *ed 4, St Louis, 1996, Mosby.)*

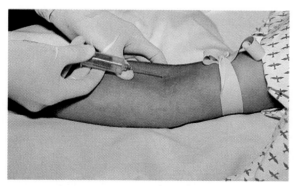

Fig. 9-17 *Inserting the needle into the vein. (From Perry AG, Potter PA:* Clinical nursing skills and techniques, *ed 4, St Louis, 1996, Mosby.)*

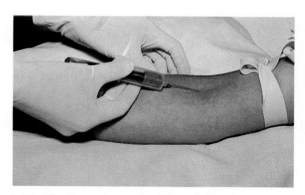

Fig. 9-18 *The Vacutainer tube fills with blood. (From Perry AG, Potter PA:* Clinical nursing skills and techniques, *ed 4, St Louis, 1996, Mosby.)*

Butterfly Method

Some people have small or weak hand veins. Other sites may be bruised from frequent venipunctures. The butterfly method is useful for such persons. The method involves using a butterfly needle (see Fig. 7-6, *B*, p. 123), a vacuum tube needle and tube holder, and vacuum tubes.

The vacuum tube needle and tube holder attach to the butterfly needle tubing. The butterfly needle is used for the venipuncture. Blood flows into the butterfly needle, into the vacuum tube needle, and into the vacuum tube. The method also allows the collection of many specimens.

BLOOD GLUCOSE TESTING

Diabetes mellitus is a chronic disease in which the pancreas fails to secrete enough insulin. Insufficient amounts of insulin prevent the body from using sugar for energy. Sugar builds up in the blood if it cannot be used. Blood glucose testing is done to measure blood sugar levels. The doctor uses the results to regulate the person's medication and diet. Inaccurate results are harmful to the person.

Complex tests are done in the laboratory. Two simple blood glucose tests are done at the bedside or in home settings. Both involve reagent strips. The blood reacts with the test area on the reagent strip. The reaction causes the test area to change color. Capillary blood is used for both tests. A skin puncture is done to obtain the specimen.

One method involves exposing the reagent strip to blood. After waiting the recommended amount of time, the blood is wiped or rinsed off the reagent strip. Then the reagent strip is compared with a color chart. The results are read and reported to the RN. You record them following facility policy. As always, follow the manufacturer's instructions for using the reagent strips.

The other method involves using a glucose meter (glucometer). A drop of blood is applied to the reagent strip. The strip is inserted into the glucose meter. The blood glucose level is displayed on the monitor. The speed with which results are displayed varies with the manufacturer. Some take as long as 2 minutes. Others take 15 seconds. Many different glucose meters are available. Always read and follow the manufacturer's instructions. Make sure you know how to use the equipment before testing blood. Also check the manufacturer's instructions for the reagent strip to use. Use only the type of reagent strip specified by the manufacturer. Otherwise you will get inaccurate results.

Also check the manufacturer's instructions about how to treat a strip before inserting it into the glucose meter.

BOX 9-1 RULES FOR BLOOD GLUCOSE TESTING

- Read the manufacturer's instructions. Make sure you understand them.
- Make sure you know how to use the equipment. Request any necessary training.
- Make sure the glucose meter was tested for accuracy. Check the testing log.
- Check the color of reagent strips. Do not use them if they are discolored.
- Check the expiration date of the reagent strips. Do not use them if the date has passed.
- Use a watch with a sweep hand to time the test. Follow the manufacturer's instructions for test times.
- Report the results immediately to the RN.
- Record the results following facility policy.
- Practice Standard Precautions.
- Follow the Bloodborne Pathogen Standard. ❈

The manufacturer requires one of the following:

- Dry-wipe—blood is wiped off the reagent strip with a cotton ball
- Wet-wash—the reagent strip is flushed with water to rinse blood off
- No-wipe—no wiping or rinsing; the reagent strip is inserted directly into the glucose meter

In facilities, glucose meters are tested daily for accuracy. Inaccurate results can harm the person. The manufacturer has specific instructions for testing the meter. Specially trained staff members perform the tests.

Accurate results are important. The rules in Box 9-1 are followed when testing blood specimens for glucose.

focus on home care Patients and families monitor blood glucose in the home setting. The person may have a routine for testing blood glucose. Ask the person how he or she does the test. Report the routine to the RN. The RN lets you follow the routine if it is safe for the person. If it is unsafe, the RN plans for patient and family teaching.

The patient keeps a record of the test results. Share the results with the person, and report them to the RN. Also record the results following agency policy.

MEASURING BLOOD GLUCOSE

PRE-PROCEDURE

1 Review the procedure with the RN.

2 Explain the procedure to the person.

3 Wash your hands.

4 Collect the following:

- Sterile lancet
- Alcohol swab
- Cotton balls
- Glucose testing meter

- Reagent strips (Make sure they are the correct ones for the meter. Check the expiration date.)
- Disposable gloves
- Paper towel
- Soap, towel, and wash basin

5 Arrange supplies on the overbed table.

6 Identify the person. Check the ID bracelet with the assignment sheet.

7 Raise the bed to a good level for body mechanics.

PROCEDURE

8 Ask the person to wash his or her hands. Provide necessary supplies and equipment.

9 Help the person assume a comfortable position.

10 Prepare the supplies:

a Open the alcohol swabs.

b Remove a reagent strip from the bottle. Place it on the paper towel. Place the cap securely on the bottle.

c Prepare the lancet.

d Turn on the glucose meter.

11 Put on the gloves.

12 Perform a skin puncture to obtain a drop of blood (see *Performing a Skin Puncture* on p. 144).

13 Wipe off the first drop of blood with a cotton ball.

14 Apply gentle pressure below the puncture site.

15 Allow a large drop of blood to form (see Fig. 9-4).

16 Hold the test area of the reagent strip close to the drop of blood.

17 Lightly touch the reagent strip to the blood drop. Do not smear the blood.

18 Set the timer on the glucose meter.

19 Set the reagent strip on the paper towel. Or follow the manufacturer's instructions.

20 Wait the length of time required by the manufacturer.

21 Apply pressure to the puncture site until bleeding stops. Use a cotton ball. If the person is able, let the person continue to apply pressure to the site.

22 Treat the reagent strip according to the manufacturer's instructions. Use the dry-wipe, wet-wash, or no-wipe method (see p. 154).

23 Insert the reagent strip into the glucose meter (Fig. 9-19, p. 156). Follow the manufacturer's instructions.

24 Read the result on the display (Fig. 9-20, p. 156). Write down the result, and tell the person the result.

25 Turn off the glucose meter.

26 Discard the lancet into the sharps container.

27 Discard the cotton balls following facility policy. (The cotton balls contain blood.)

28 Remove and discard the gloves.

Continued

MEASURING BLOOD GLUCOSE—CONT'D

POST-PROCEDURE

29 Help the person to a comfortable position.

30 Make sure the call bell is within reach.

31 Raise or lower bed rails as instructed by the RN.

32 Lower the bed to its lowest horizontal position.

33 Unscreen the person.

34 Discard used supplies. Clean and return the bath basin to its proper place.

35 Follow facility policy for soiled linen.

36 Wash your hands.

37 Report the following to the RN immediately:
- The time the specimen was collected
- The test results
- The site used
- How the person tolerated the procedure
- Other observations or patient complaints

38 Record the result following facility policy.

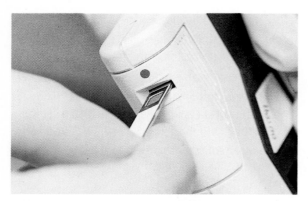

Fig. 9-19 *Inserting the reagent strip into the glucose meter.* (From Elkin MK, Perry AG, Potter PA: Nursing interventions and clinical skills, St Louis, 1996, Mosby.)

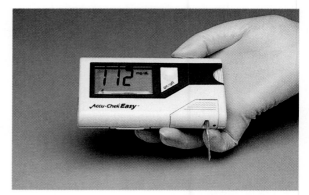

Fig. 9-20 *Reading the result on the glucose meter display.* (From Elkin MK, Perry AG, Potter PA: Nursing interventions and clinical skills, St Louis, 1996, Mosby.)

SUMMARY

Blood tests are important in detecting and treating disease. They are common diagnostic tools. Most tests are done in the laboratory. Blood specimens are obtained by venipuncture. Simple blood tests like blood glucose testing are done at the bedside or in home settings. Capillary blood is used. It is obtained by skin puncture. Accuracy is an important part of blood glucose testing.

Sterile needles and lancets are used to obtain blood specimens. You must not touch the needle or lancet.

After obtaining the specimen, the needle or lancet is discarded into a sharps container. This prevents needle sticks and contact with the person's blood. Always practice Standard Precautions and follow the Bloodborne Pathogen Standard when collecting and testing blood specimens. You must protect yourself and others from bloodborne diseases.

Venipunctures and skin punctures are uncomfortable. Performing these procedures quickly and efficiently promotes the person's comfort.

REVIEW QUESTIONS

Circle the best *answer.*

1 A tourniquet is
   a A swelling that contains blood
   b A blood test
   c A device to control bleeding
   d A short, disposable blade

2 The most common site for a skin puncture is
   a The earlobe
   b The heal
   c The thumb
   d A fingertip

3 You inspect a skin puncture site. You avoid the site if it is
   a Calloused
   b Swollen or bruised
   c Scarred
   d All of the above

4 To avoid painful skin punctures, puncture the fingertip
   a At the side of the fingertip
   b In the center of the fingertip
   c In the fleshy part of the fingertip
   d All of the above

5 You perform a skin puncture. The first drop of blood is
   a Saved
   b Wiped off with a cotton ball
   c Tested in case you cannot get another drop
   d Rinsed off with water

6 After puncturing the skin, the lancet is
   a Discarded into the sharps container
   b Sterilized for reuse
   c Discarded with other supplies
   d Capped

7 Blood specimens are labeled at the nurses' station.
   a True
   b False

8 You are to perform a venipuncture. What veins should you use?
   a Hand veins
   b Foot veins
   c Veins in the antecubital space
   d All of the above

9 You are selecting a vein for a venipucture. The vein should
   a Rebound after palpating it
   b Be narrow
   c Be sclerosed
   d Roll easily

10 The needle and syringe method is used to obtain a blood specimen. Which is *true?*
   a The needle is capped. The needle and syringe are sent to the laboratory.
   b The needle is discarded. The syringe is capped and sent to the laboratory.
   c The blood is transferred from the syringe to a test tube.
   d Blood is collected in Vacutainers.

11 You are going to test blood glucose with a glucose meter. Which is *false?*
   a The blood specimen is obtained by venipuncture.
   b The manufacturer's instructions must be followed.
   c The expiration date on the reagent strips is checked.
   d The results are immediately reported to the RN.

12 The manufacturer requires the dry-wipe method for reagent strips. This means that
   a Blood is rinsed off before inserting the reagent strip into the glucose meter.
   b The first drop of blood from the skin puncture is wiped off with a cotton ball.
   c Blood is wiped off with a cotton ball before inserting the reagent strip into the glucose meter.
   d The reagent strip is inserted directly into the glucose meter.

Answers to these questions are on p. 179

10 Obtaining an Electrocardiogram

OBJECTIVES

- Define the key terms in this chapter
- Explain why electrocardiograms are obtained
- Describe the structures and function of the heart
- Explain the conduction system of the heart
- Identify the normal waves of an electrocardiogram
- Locate the sites for limb leads and chest leads
- Identify the functions of the electrocardiograph
- Describe electrocardiograph paper
- Calculate the heart rate using a 6-second strip
- Explain how to prepare the person for an electrocardiogram
- Obtain an electrocardiogram
- Know the dysrhythmias that are life-threatening

KEY TERMS

arrhythmia Without *(a)* a rhythm

artifact Interference on the electrocardiogram

dysrhythmia An abnormal *(dys)* rhythm

electrocardiogram A recording *(gram)* of the electrical activity *(electro)* of the heart *(cardio);* ECG or EKG

electrocardiograph An instrument *(graph)* that records the electrical activity *(electro)* of the heart *(cardio)*

lead A pair of electrodes; electrical activity is recorded between the electrodes

An **electrocardiogram** (ECG or EKG) is a recording *(gram)* of the electrical activity *(electro)* of the heart *(cardio)*. Changes occur in the ECG when the heart muscle is damaged. The doctor can locate the area of heart damage by studying the ECG. An irregular heart rhythm is detected by taking a pulse. However, an ECG is required to identify the type of irregular rhythm.

Therefore doctors order ECGs for persons with chest pain, pain in the upper arms, and irregular heart rhythms. Persons with abnormal blood pressures also require ECGs. These signs and symptoms may signal heart disease.

ECGs also are done before surgery. This is to make sure that the person does not go to surgery with a heart problem. Fitness tests and health physical examinations often include ECGs. By detecting heart problems early, life-threatening heart diseases can be prevented.

Obtaining ECGs is commonly done by assistive personnel. As with other procedures, make sure that:

- Your state allows you to perform the procedure

- The procedure is in your job description

- You have the necessary education and training

- You know how to use the facility's equipment

- An RN is available to answer questions and supervise you

THE HEART

The heart is a muscle. It pumps blood through the blood vessels to the tissues and cells. The heart lies in the middle to lower part of the chest cavity toward the left side (Fig. 10-1, p. 160). The heart is hollow and has three layers (Fig. 10-2, p. 160):

- The *pericardium* is the outer layer. It is a thin sac covering the heart.

- The *myocardium* is the second layer. This layer is the thick, muscular portion of the heart.

- The *endocardium* is the inner layer. It is the membrane lining the inner surface of the heart.

The heart has four chambers (see Fig. 10-2). Upper chambers receive blood and are called the *atria*. The *right atrium* receives blood from body tissues. The *left atrium* receives blood from the lungs. Lower chambers are called *ventricles*. Ventricles pump blood. The *right ventricle* pumps blood to the lungs for oxygen. The *left ventricle* pumps blood to all parts of the body.

There are two phases of heart action. During *diastole,* the resting phase, heart chambers fill with blood. The heart relaxes during this phase. During *systole,* the working phase, the heart contracts. Blood is pumped through the blood vessels when the heart contracts. Systole and diastole make up the *cardiac cycle.*

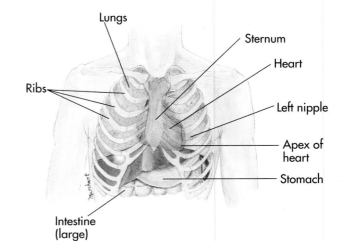

Fig. 10-1 *Location of the heart in the chest cavity.*

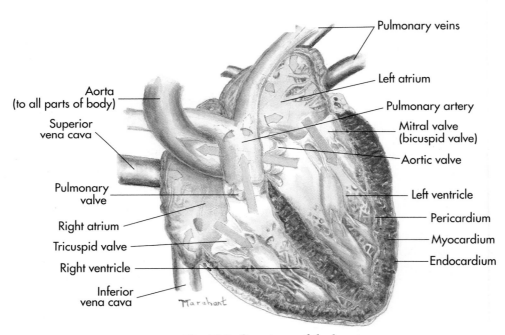

Fig. 10-2 *Structures of the heart.*

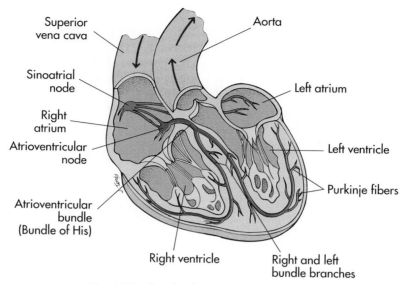

Fig. 10-3 *Conduction system of the heart.*

Conduction System

The conduction system controls the cardiac cycle. The heart muscle must relax (fill with blood) and contract (pump blood) in a coordinated fashion. Otherwise cells do not get enough blood and oxygen.

To coordinate the cardiac cycle, the heart's muscle fibers are linked together. An electrical impulse starts in the wall of the right atrium. It passes through (is conducted or transmitted to) muscle fibers in the right and left atria, causing the atria to contract. Then the impulse moves to the ventricles, causing the ventricles to contract. For every heartbeat, an electrical impulse is conducted through the heart.

Four structures in the heart wall make up the conduction system (Fig. 10-3). They are the sinoatrial node, atrioventricular node, atrioventricular bundle, and the Purkinje fibers:

- *Sinoatrial node (SA node)* starts the impulse in the right atrium. The SA node is also called the *pacemaker*. It sets the pace (beat) of the heart.

- The electrical impulse travels from SA node to the right and left atria.

- The right and left atria contract as the impulse travels through them. Blood is pumped to the ventricles.

- The electrical impulse reaches the *atrioventricular node (AV node)*. It is located at the bottom of the right atrium (*atrio*) near the right ventricle (*ventricular*).

- The impulse travels through the AV node to the *atrioventricular bundle (AV bundle)* in the wall separating the right and left ventricles. (The AV bundle is also called the *bundle of His*.)

- The AV bundle has right and left branches that extend to all parts of the ventricular wall. The *right bundle branch* conducts the impulse to the right ventricle. The *left bundle branch* conducts the impulse to the left ventricle.

- *Purkinje fibers* branch into the myocardium (heart muscle) from the right and left bundle branches. When the impulse reaches the ventricular muscle, the ventricles contract.

- After contracting, the ventricles relax.

Areas outside the SA node can act as a pacemaker. That is, they can start an impulse. This causes an irregular heart beat. Some rhythms are life-threatening.

Blocks can occur in the conduction system. A block prevents the impulse from traveling through the conduction system in a normal manner. Blocks also can be life-threatening.

THE ELECTROCARDIOGRAM

ECGs record the electrical activity of the conduction system. The electrical activity is recorded in waves. The waves give the cardiac cycle a distinct appearance. Each wave represents electrical activity in a certain part of the heart. The *P wave*, *QRS complex*, and *T wave* are the major parts of the cardiac cycle. Figure 10-4 shows the electrical activity in the cardiac cycle.

If a problem occurs in a part of the conduction system, the wave representing that part appears abnormal. Problems can occur in any part of the conduction system. ECG changes also occur if the heart muscle is damaged. By studying the ECG, the doctor determines the site of the problem in the conduction system or the area of heart muscle damage.

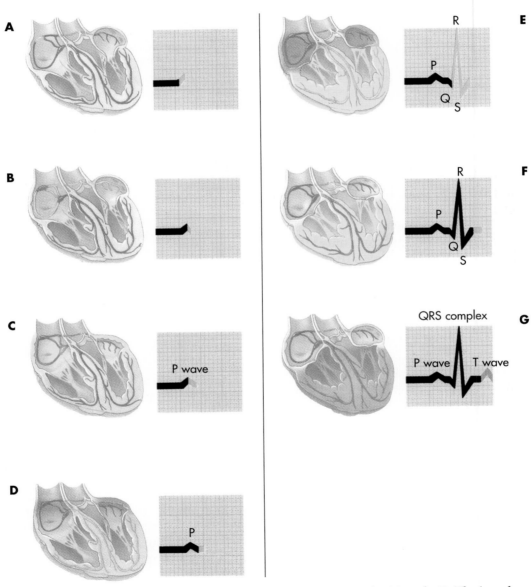

Fig. 10-4 *Electrical activity in the heart. **A,** The impulse starts in the SA node. **B,** The impulse spreads to the right and left atria. **C,** The atria contract. The P wave is formed. **D,** The impulse reaches the AV node and the AV bundle. The atria relax. **E,** The ventricles contract. The QRS complex forms. **F,** The ventricles start to relax. **G,** The ventricles relax. The T wave forms. (From Thibodeau GA, Patton KT: Structure and function of the human body, ed 10, St Louis, 1997, Mosby.)*

ECG Leads

The cardiac cycle involves electrical currents passing through the heart. The currents travel in many directions. These currents also are conducted to the body's surface. The currents can be detected with electrodes placed on the body's surface. Electrical activity is recorded between two electrodes. Each pair of electrodes is called a **lead.**

The standard ECG involves 12 leads. It is called a *12-lead ECG.* The heart's electrical activity is recorded from different directions. The cardiac cycle (P wave, QRS complex, and T wave) appears different from each of the 12 directions (Fig. 10-5).

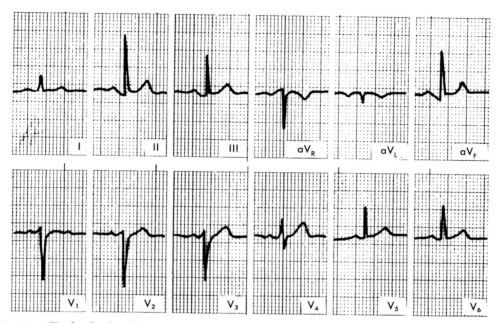

Fig. 10-5 *Twelve leads of the electrocardiogram. (From Kinney M, Packa D, Andreoli K, Zipes D:* Comprehensive cardiac care, *ed 8, St Louis, 1996, Mosby.)*

Limb leads Electrical current from the heart travels to the arms and legs—the limbs. Electrodes are attached to each limb. The 6 limb leads involve 3 standard limb leads and 3 augmented limb leads.

The *standard limb leads* are numbered with Roman numerals. They also are called *bipolar limb leads*. They measure electrical activity between two *(bi)* points *(poles)* (Fig. 10-6):

- Lead I—records electrical activity between the right arm (RA) and left arm (LA)

- Lead II—records electrical activity between the right arm (RA) and left leg (LL)

- Lead III—records electrical activity between the left arm (LA) and left leg (LL)

The *augmented unipolar limb leads* produce larger wave forms that are easier to read. (To *augment* means to increase or enlarge.) They record the heart's electrical activity from one *(uni)* limb lead *(pole)* to the midpoint of the two other leads (Fig. 10-7). These three leads are called aV_R, aV_L, and aV_F (the letter *a* means *augmented*; The letter *V* stands for *unipolar*):

- aV_R—records electrical activity from the right arm (R) to the midpoint between the electrodes on the left arm and left leg

- aV_L—records electrical activity from the left arm (L) to the midpoint between the electrodes on the right arm and left leg

- aV_F—records electrical activity from the left leg (F) to the midpoint between the electrodes on the right arm and left arm

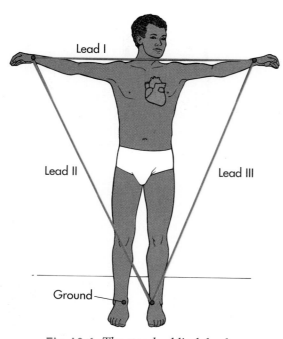

Fig. 10-6 *The standard limb leads.*

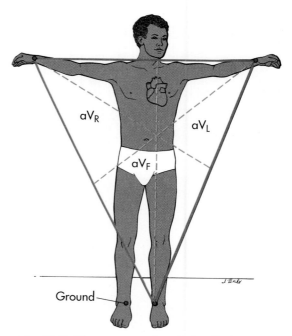

Fig. 10-7 *The augmented unipolar limb leads.*

Chest leads Chest leads also are called *precordial leads.* Precordial means in front of *(pre)* the heart *(cor).* These leads are placed at 6 different sites on the chest (Fig. 10-8). The sites are over the heart. The 6 chest leads are numbered V_1 through V_6. (The V stands for unipolar).

The chest leads are placed as follows:

- V_1—at the fourth intercostal space on the right side of the sternum. *Intercostal* means between *(inter)* the ribs *(costal).* The fourth intercostal space is between the third and fourth ribs

- V_2—at the fourth intercostal space on the left side of the sternum

- V_3—halfway between V_2 and V_4

- V_4—at the fifth intercostal space at the midclavicular line. The fifth intercostal space is between the fifth and sixth ribs. *Midclavicular* means in the middle *(mid)* of the *clavicle.* To find the midclavicular line, find the clavicle. Then find the middle of the clavicle. Draw an imaginary line down to the fifth intercostal space. (This is usually below the left nipple.)

- V_5—at the level of V_4 and the anterior axillary line. The *anterior axillary* line is in front of *(anterior)* the underarm *(axillary)*

- V_6—at the level of V_4 and the midaxillary line. *Midaxillary* means the middle *(mid)* of the underarm *(axillary)*

The Electrocardiograph

The **electrocardiograph** is an instrument *(graph)* that records the electrical activity *(electro)* of the heart *(cardio).* The machine is portable and is brought to the person's bedside when an ECG is ordered (Fig. 10-9).

The ECG machine senses the heart's electrical activity from the electrodes. Cables attach the electrodes on the person's body to the machine. The machine processes electrical activity. Then it displays the activity in the form of a graph (Fig. 10-10).

All ECG machines sense, process, and display the heart's electrical activity. You will learn how to use the ECG machines in your facility. Always follow the manufacturer's instructions.

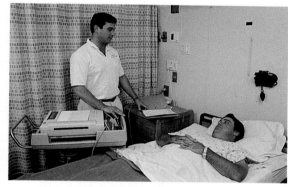

Fig. 10-9 *The electrocardiograph is brought to the person's bedside.*

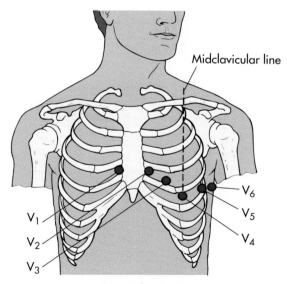

Fig. 10-8 *The chest leads.*

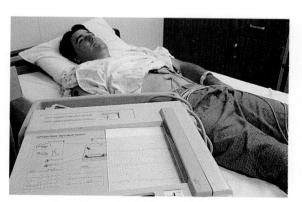

Fig. 10-10 *The electrocardiograph displays a recording of the heart's electrical activity.*

Electrocardiograph paper Electrocardiograph paper is divided into squares (Fig. 10-11). The larger squares (heavy black lines) are divided into smaller squares (light black lines).

Moving vertically (from bottom to top), the squares represent *voltage*. Voltage is a measure of electrical force. The greater the force coming from the heart muscle, the higher the wave formed on the ECG. When studying the ECG, the doctor looks at the height of the waves in each lead. Depending on the lead, the wave may be above the baseline or below it.

Moving horizontally (from left to right), the squares represent *time*. Each small square represents 0.04 second. Note that each large square has five small squares. Therefore each large square represents 0.20 second (0.04 second × 5 = 0.20 second).

The P wave, QRS complex, and T wave of the cardiac cycle normally occur in a certain pattern (Fig. 10-12). Normal time intervals occur between the P wave and QRS complex (PR interval) and between the QRS complex and the T wave (QT interval). Abnormal patterns and time intervals signal heart problems.

The ECG paper also is marked along the top white margin (Fig. 10-13). The notches occur in 1-second intervals. The indicator lines are longer or darker every 3 second. Note that there are 5 large boxes between two notches. Remember, each large box represents 0.20 second. Therefore 5 large boxes represent 1 second (0.20 second × 5 = 1 second). These notches are useful for estimating the person's heart rate. Simply count the number of R waves within a 6-second strip. Multiply that number by 10. In Figure 10-14, the heart rate is 70.

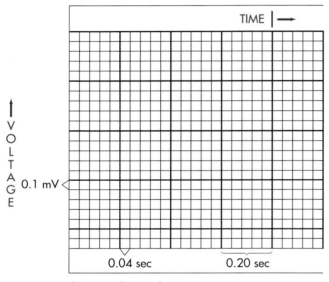

Fig. 10-11 *Electrocardiograph paper. (From Phipps WJ, Sands J, Lehman MK, Cassmeyer V:* Medical-surgical nursing: concepts and clinical practice, *ed 5, St Louis, 1995, Mosby.)*

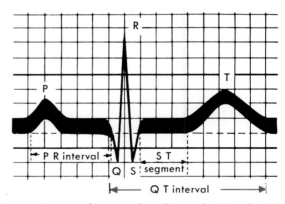

Fig. 10-12 *Pattern of a normal cardiac cycle. Note the PR interval and the ST segment. (From Kinney M, Packa D, Andreoli K, Zipes D:* Comprehensive cardiac care, *ed 8, St Louis, 1996, Mosby.)*

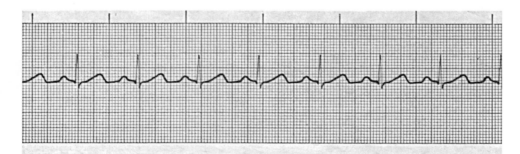

Fig. 10-13 *Indicator lines on ECG paper. Each short line represents 1 second. The longer lines represent 3 seconds. (From Atwood S, Stanton C, Storey J:* Introduction to basic cardiac dysrhythmias, *ed 2, St Louis, 1996, Mosby.)*

Artifact Sometimes interference occurs on the ECG. This is called **artifact.** P waves, QRS complexes, and T waves are not clear and distinct (Fig. 10-15, *A* and *B*). Sometimes the baseline looks fuzzy (Fig. 10-15, *C*). Poorly connected or loose electrodes can cause artifact. Excess chest hair and sweating can interfere with electrode contact with the skin. Broken cable wires also cause artifact. So can patient movements such as shivering and rapid breathing. Do not confuse artifact with abnormal rhythms (see p. 170). If in doubt, call for the RN.

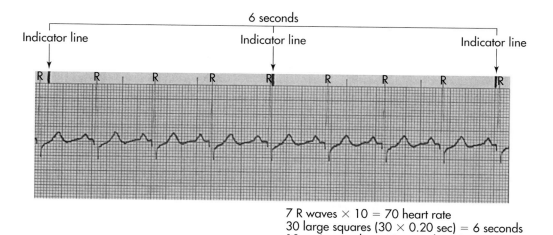

7 R waves × 10 = 70 heart rate
30 large squares (30 × 0.20 sec) = 6 seconds
10 × 6 seconds = 60 seconds or 1 minute

Fig. 10-14 *Estimating the heart rate with a 6-second strip. Seven R waves × 10 = 70 beats per minute.* *(From Atwood S, Stanton C, Storey J:* Introduction to basic cardiac dysrhythmias, *ed 2, St Louis, 1996, Mosby.)*

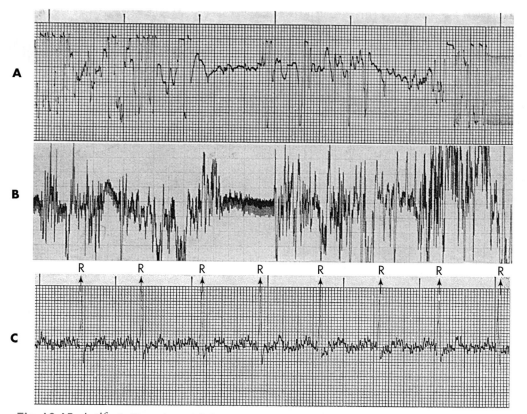

Fig. 10-15 *Artifact. (From Atwood S, Stanton C, Storey J:* Introduction to basic cardiac dysrhythmias, *ed 2, St Louis, 1996, Mosby.)*

Obtaining an ECG

The person must be mentally and physically prepared for an ECG. Often ECGs are done when the person is experiencing chest pain. The person may be having a heart attack. The person is frightened and in pain and may have difficulty breathing. This life-threatening situation requires prompt action and a calm manner.

The RN tells you when to obtain an ECG. Sometimes ECGs are ordered *stat*. Stat is an abbreviation for the Latin word *statim*, which means immediately.

The RN explains the procedure to the person and why it is necessary. As you perform the procedure, you also explain what you are going to do. This helps calm the person.

The supine position is preferred for the ECG. However, persons with severe chest pain and difficulty breathing may find the supine position uncomfortable. Ask the RN how you should position the person.

The electrodes must have good contact with the skin for a clear recording. Skin preparation is important. Electrode sites are wiped with alcohol. This removes skin oils and perspiration. Allow the sites to dry before applying the electrodes.

Excessive chest and body hair can prevent good skin-electrode contact. Shaving electrode sites is often necessary. Explain to the person why you need to shave these sites. Be careful not to nick or cut the skin. Wear gloves when shaving to avoid possible contact with blood. Standard Precautions and the Bloodborne Pathogen Standard are followed.

You must call for the RN immediately if the person develops problems during the ECG. Stay with the person until the RN arrives. Then follow the RN's instructions. Call for the RN immediately if the person has any of the following:

- Chest pain
- Pain in the jaw or down the arms
- Dyspnea or shortness of breath
- Changes in mental function
- Tachycardia (calculate a 6-second strip)
- Bradycardia (calculate a 6-second strip)
- Abnormal beats (see p. 170).
- An abnormal rhythm (see p. 170)

OBTAINING AN ECG

PRE-PROCEDURE

1 Review the procedure with the RN.
2 Explain the procedure to the person.
3 Wash your hands.
4 Collect the following:
   - Electrocardiograph
   - Electrodes
   - Alcohol wipes
   - Razor
   - Towel
   - Disposable gloves
   - Requisition slip

5 Review the manufacturer's instructions for the ECG machine.
6 Arrange equipment in a convenient location in the person's room.
7 Identify the person. Check the ID bracelet with the requisition slip.
8 Provide for privacy.
9 Raise the bed to the best level for good body mechanics.
10 Assist the person with elimination needs. This helps the person relax. Clean and return equipment to its proper place. Remove gloves, and wash your hands. (The person may be seriously ill. The person's condition may not allow time for this step.)

OBTAINING AN ECG—CONT'D

PROCEDURE

11 Measure the person's vital signs. Make a note of them.

12 Position the person supine.

13 Expose only the person's chest, arms, and legs.

14 Determine if you will need to shave any electrode sites.

15 Shave electrode sites as needed:

  a Place a towel under the site.

  b Put on disposable gloves.

  c Shave the site.

  d Move the towel to the next site. Avoid getting hair on bed linens.

  e Shave that site.

  f Repeats Steps 15 d and e as necessary.

  g Remove and discard the gloves.

16 Clean the electrode sites with the alcohol wipes.

17 Allow electrode sites to dry.

18 Apply the electrodes to the chest, arms, and legs (see Figs. 10-6 and 10-8).

19 Connect the cables from the machine to the electrodes (Fig. 10-16).

20 Plug the ECG machine into a wall outlet.

21 Ask the person to lie still. Remind the person not to talk or to cross his or her legs.

22 Obtain an 8- to 12-inch tracing of each lead. Call for the RN if you see any abnormal patterns (see p. 170).

23 Turn off the ECG machine.

24 Tear the tracing off the machine.

25 Label the tracing with the person's identifying information: full name, ID number, room and bed number, and age. Also note the date and time.

26 Disconnect the cables.

27 Remove the electrodes.

28 Cover the person.

POST-PROCEDURE

29 Make sure the person is comfortable.

30 Place the call bell within reach.

31 Raise or lower bed rails as instructed by the RN.

32 Lower the bed to its lowest horizontal position.

33 Unscreen the person.

34 Discard used supplies. Follow facility policy for soiled linen.

35 Return the ECG machine to its proper location.

36 Show the ECG to the RN. Report any observations or patient complaints.

37 Take or send the ECG and requisition slip to the appropriate department.

38 Wash your hands.

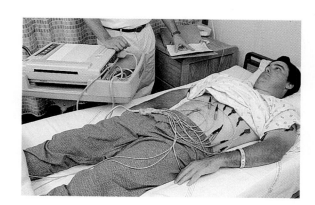

Fig. 10-16 Cables are connected from the machine to the electrodes.

DYSRHYTHMIAS

A **dysrhythmia** is an abnormal *(dys)* rhythm. The term *arrhythmia* is often used. **Arrhythmia** means without *(a)* a rhythm. The doctor or RN studies the ECG for dysrhythmias. Treatment depends on the cause and type of dysrhythmia.

Some dysrhythmias are life-threatening. Immediate action must be taken. If you see anything abnormal on a tracing, you must call for the RN immediately. Figures 10-13 and 10-14 show normal rhythms. That is, QRS complexes occur at regular intervals. The P waves and T waves appear normal. These are normal sinus rhythms. That is, the rhythm starts in the sinoatrial node (SA node) and passes through the conduction system normally. Figures 10-17 through 10-32 show some dysrhythmias that must be reported to the RN immediately:

- *Sinus tachycardia*—The heart rate is rapid (Fig. 10-17). Impulses start in the SA node.

- *Sinus bradycardia*—The heart rate is slow (Fig. 10-18). Impulses start in the SA node.

- *Premature atrial contraction (PAC)*—The SA node sends out an impulse early (Fig. 10-19).

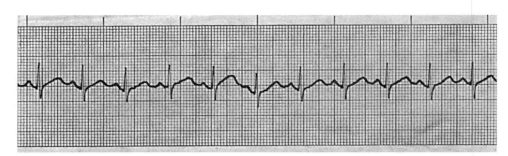

Fig. 10-17 *Sinus tachycardia. The heart rate is 110. (From Atwood S, Stanton C, Storey J:* Introduction to basic cardiac dysrhythmias, *ed 2, St Louis, 1996, Mosby.)*

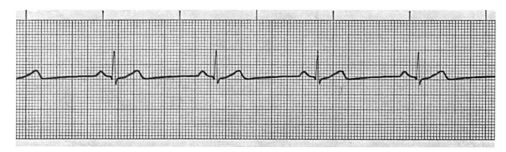

Fig. 10-18 *Sinus bradycardia. The heart rate is 40. (From Atwood S, Stanton C, Storey J:* Introduction to basic cardiac dysrhythmias, *ed 2, St Louis, 1996, Mosby.)*

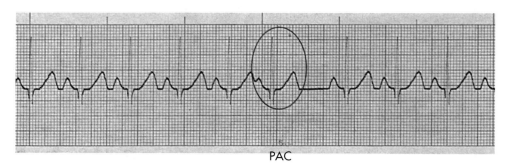

PAC

Fig. 10-19 *Premature atrial contraction (PAC). (From Atwood S, Stanton C, Storey J:* Introduction to basic cardiac dysrhythmias, *ed 2, St Louis, 1996, Mosby.)*

- *Paroxysmal atrial tachycardia (PAT)*—A normal rhythm suddenly turns into tachycardia. Bursts (paroxysms) of tachycardia occur. The tachycardia stops suddenly (Fig. 10-20).

- *Atrial flutter*—Impulses start in the atria at a rapid rate. The ventricles do not respond to every impulse (Fig. 10-21). There are more P waves (flutter or F waves) than QRS complexes. QRS complexes occur at regular intervals. The person's pulse is regular.

- *Atrial fibrillation*—Impulses start in the atria at multiple sites. There are no P waves. Impulses are conducted to the ventricles at irregular intervals (Fig. 10-22). QRS complexes occur at irregular intervals. Therefore the pulse is irregular. The atria quiver, not contract. Blood is not pumped from the atria to the ventricles in normal amounts. Therefore the ventricles pump inadequate amounts of blood to the rest of the body.

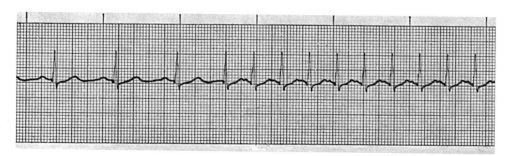

Fig. 10-20 *Paroxysmal atrial tachycardia (PAT).* *(From Atwood S, Stanton C, Storey J:* Introduction to basic cardiac dysrhythmias, *ed 2, St Louis, 1996, Mosby.)*

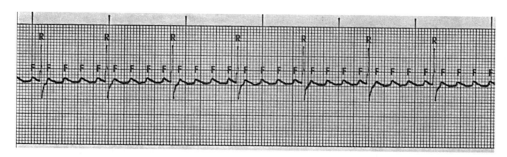

Fig. 10-21 *Atrial flutter. Note the F waves.* *(From Atwood S, Stanton C, Storey J:* Introduction to basic cardiac dysrhythmias, *ed 2, St Louis, 1996, Mosby.)*

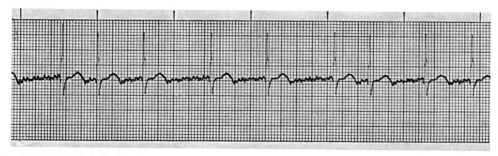

Fig. 10-22 *Atrial fibrillation. No P waves occur, and the rhythm is irregular.* *(From Atwood S, Stanton C, Storey J:* Introduction to basic cardiac dysrhythmias, *ed 2, St Louis, 1996, Mosby.)*

- *Junctional rhythms*—Impulses start in the AV node. There are no P waves (Fig. 10-23). Junctional rhythms can occur at normal or slow rates.

- *Third-degree heart block*—The impulse is blocked between the atria and ventricles (Fig. 10-24). The impulse cannot reach the ventricles. The ventricles must create their own impulses. P waves appear but are not related to the QRS complexes. The QRS complexes are wider than normal. The heart rate is very slow. **This is a life-threatening dysrythmia.**

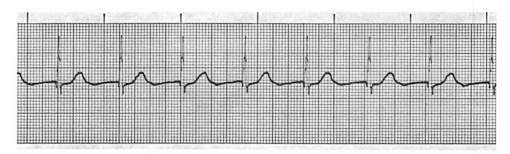

Fig. 10-23 *Junctional rhythm. No P waves. (From Atwood S, Stanton C, Storey J:* Introduction to basic cardiac dysrhythmias, *ed 2, St Louis, 1996, Mosby.)*

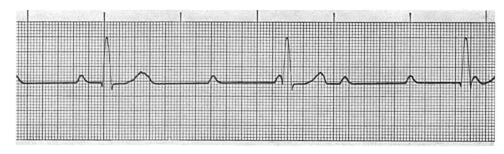

Fig. 10-24 *Third-degree heart block. The atrial rate (P waves) is faster than the ventricular rate.* *(From Atwood S, Stanton C, Storey J:* Introduction to basic cardiac dysrhythmias, *ed 2, St Louis, 1996, Mosby.)*

- *Premature ventricular contraction (PVC)*—The impulse is created in the ventricles. It occurs earlier than the next regular beat. The QRS complex is wide and bizarre (Fig. 10-25). *Unifocal PVCs* come from one *(uni)* site *(focal)*. They all look the same. *Multifocal PVCs* are created in many *(multi)* sites *(focal)* as in Figure 10-26. *Bigeminy* is when every second *(bi)* complex is a PVC (Fig. 10-27). With *trigeminy,* every third *(tri)* complex is a PVC. *(Geminus* means twin.) Two PVCs can occur in a row (Fig. 10-28, p. 174). They can be unifocal or multifocal and are called *coupled PVCs.* A *run of ventricular tachycardia* is several PVCs in a row (Fig. 10-29, p. 174). The rhythm returns to normal. PVCs mean that the heart muscle is irritable. **PVCs are life-threatening.**

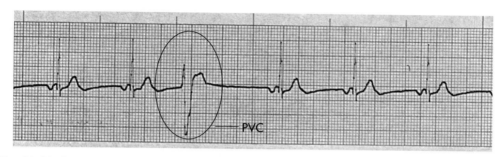

Fig. 10-25 *Premature ventricular contraction (PVC). (From Atwood S, Stanton C, Storey J:* Introduction to basic cardiac dysrhythmias, *ed 2, St Louis, 1996, Mosby.)*

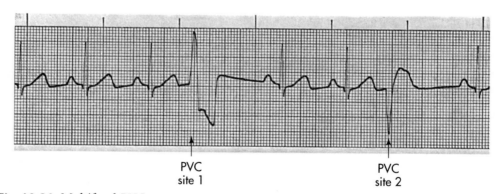

Fig. 10-26 *Multifocal PVCs. (From Atwood S, Stanton C, Storey J:* Introduction to basic cardiac dysrhythmias, *ed 2, St Louis, 1996, Mosby.)*

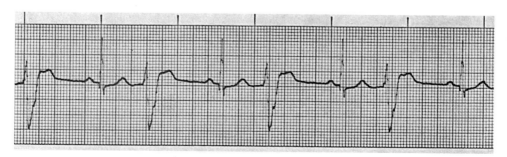

Fig. 10-27 *Bigeminy. (From Atwood S, Stanton C, Storey J:* Introduction to basic cardiac dysrhythmias, *ed 2, St Louis, 1996, Mosby.)*

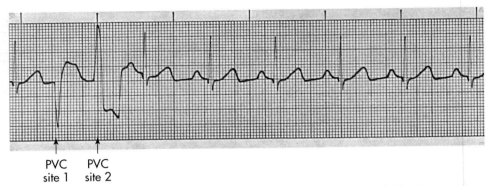

PVC   PVC
site 1 site 2

Fig. 10-28 *Coupled PVCs. Two PVCs occur in a row. The PVCs are multifocal.* *(From Atwood S, Stanton C, Storey J:* Introduction to basic cardiac dysrhythmias, *ed 2, St Louis, 1996, Mosby.)*

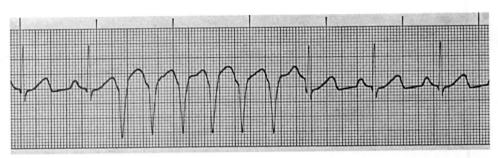

Fig. 10-29 *Run of ventricular tachycardia.* *(From Atwood S, Stanton C, Storey J:* Introduction to basic cardiac dysrhythmias, *ed 2, St Louis, 1996, Mosby.)*

- *Ventricular tachycardia (VT)*—Impulses start in the ventricles. The heart rate can range from 40 to 250 per minute. QRS complexes are wide and bizarre. The rhythm looks like a series of PVCs (Fig. 10-30). **Ventricular tachycardia is life-threatening. If not corrected, it progresses to ventricular fibrillation.**

- *Ventricular fibrillation (V Fib)*—Impulses start from multiple sites in the ventricles. P waves and QRS complexes are not present (Fig. 10-31). The ventricles quiver, not contract. **Ventricular fibrillation is deadly. The person is in cardiac arrest.**

- *Asystole*—No *(a)* contraction *(systole)* occurs. No electrical activity occurs in the heart (Fig. 10-32). **Asystole is deadly. The person is in cardiac arrest.**

Always look at the person when you see ECG patterns similar to ventricular tachycardia (see Fig. 10-30), ventricular fibrillation (see Fig. 10-31), and asystole (see Fig. 10-32). Check to see if the person is moving and breathing. Disconnected cables, improper electrode placement, and patient movements can cause similar patterns (see p. 167). Initiate your facility's life support procedures if the person:

- Is unresponsive

- Is not breathing

- Has no pulse

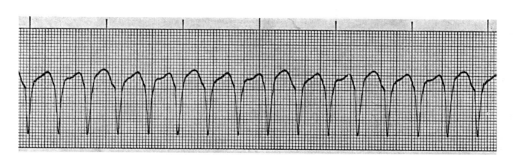

Fig. 10-30 *Ventricular tachycardia (VT). The rate is 160. (From Atwood S, Stanton C, Storey J:* Introduction to basic cardiac dysrhythmias, *ed 2, St Louis, 1996, Mosby.)*

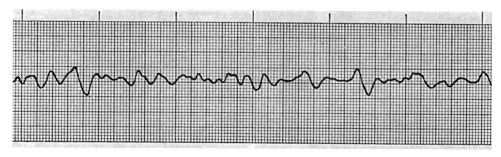

Fig. 10-31 *Ventricular fibrillation—no P waves or QRS complexes. (From Atwood S, Stanton C, Storey J:* Introduction to basic cardiac dysrhythmias, *ed 2, St Louis, 1996, Mosby.)*

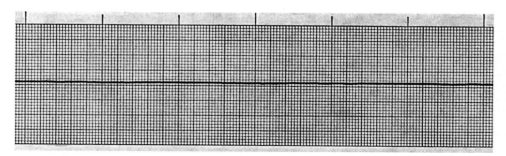

Fig. 10-32 *Asystole. (From Atwood S, Stanton C, Storey J:* Introduction to basic cardiac dysrhythmias, *ed 2, St Louis, 1996, Mosby.)*

SUMMARY

ECGs give important information about the electrical activity of the heart. They reveal areas of heart muscle damage and allow dysrhythmia identification. The information is used to plan appropriate treatment. Often life-threatening events are prevented.

When obtaining an ECG, a clear tracing is important. The person must lie still, and electrodes need good skin contact. Always explain the procedure to the person. Knowing what to expect helps to calm a person. This helps the person lie still. Clean electrode sites with alcohol to remove skin oils and perspiration. If necessary, shave body hair at the sites. Make sure you shave only a small area.

ECGs are often done during emergency situations. A calm, professional manner is important. Always be alert for life-threatening dysrhythmias. Do not try to identify the dysrhythmia. If you see something abnormal, call for the RN immediately. Also call for the RN immediately if you observe signs and symptoms of patient distress (see p. 168).

REVIEW QUESTIONS

Circle the best answer.

1 The recording of the electrical activity of the heart is an
  a Electrocardiograph
  b Electrocardiogram
  c Arrhythmia
  d Electrode

2 The muscular portion of the heart is called the
  a Pericardium
  b Myocardium
  c Endocardium
  d Dyscardium

3 The heart muscle contracts during
  a Systole
  b Diastole
  c Fibrillation
  d Conduction

4 In normal rhythms, the impulse is created in the
  a SA node
  b AV node
  c Bundle of His
  d Purkinje fibers

5 The normal ECG has the following waves *except*
  a P waves
  b QRS complexes
  c T waves
  d F waves

6 The standard ECG involves
  a 3 leads
  b 6 leads
  c 12 leads
  d Unipolar leads

7 The chest leads also are called
  a Precordial leads
  b Limb leads
  c Augmented limb leads
  d Bipolar leads

8 To estimate the heart rate with an ECG tracing, you need a
  a 3-second strip
  b 6-second strip
  c 3-inch strip
  d 6-inch strip

9 Before applying electrodes to the skin, electrode sites are cleaned
  a By shaving
  b With soap and water
  c With alcohol wipes
  d With water

10 A person develops chest pain during an ECG. What should you do?
  a Take the person's vital signs.
  b Ask about other symptoms.
  c Continue taking the ECG.
  d Call for the RN.

11 Which dysrhythmia is not life-threatening?
  a Atrial flutter
  b Ventricular tachycardia
  c Ventricular fibrillation
  d Third-degree heart block

12 The ECG tracing appears to show asystole. What should you do?
  a Call for the RN.
  b Start life support procedures.
  c Continue taking the ECG.
  d Check to see if the person is moving and breathing.

Answers to these questions are on p. 179

ANSWERS TO REVIEW QUESTIONS

Chapter 1
Assistive Personnel

1 True
2 False
3 True
4 True
5 False
6 False
7 False
8 c
9 d
10 c
11 c
12 a
13 b
14 a
15 a
16 a
17 b
18 a
19 c
20 b
21 a
22 b
23 a
24 a
25 b
26 c
27 d

Chapter 2
Surgical Asepsis

1 False
2 True
3 True
4 False
5 True
6 True
7 False
8 True
9 True
10 False
11 True
12 True
13 False
14 True

Chapter 3
Assisting with Wound Care

1 b
2 c
3 a
4 a
5 a
6 b
7 a
8 d
9 c
10 c
11 d

12 a
13 a
14 c

Chapter 4
Oxygen Needs

1 a
2 c
3 c
4 b
5 d
6 c
7 d
8 a
9 b
10 a
11 b
12 d
13 b
14 d
15 d
16 c
17 a
18 a
19 c
20 b
21 b
22 d
23 b
24 c
25 d

Chapter 5
Urinary Elimination

1 b
2 c
3 a
4 a
5 c
6 a
7 c
8 b
9 a
10 d
11 a
12 a

Chapter 6
Enteral Nutrition

1 a
2 b
3 d
4 b
5 d
6 d
7 a
8 b
9 c
10 True
11 False

12 False
13 True
14 False
15 True

Chapter 7
Assisting with Intravenous Therapy

1 d
2 b
3 b
4 d
5 d
6 b
7 a
8 b
9 c
10 a

Chapter 8
Assisting with Blood Administration

1 c
2 a
3 d
4 b
5 c
6 d
7 c
8 a
9 b
10 a

Chapter 9
Collecting and Testing Blood Specimens

1 c
2 d
3 d
4 a
5 b
6 a
7 b
8 c
9 a
10 c
11 a
12 c

Chapter 10
Obtaining an Electrocardiogram

1 b
2 b
3 a
4 a
5 d
6 c
7 a
8 b
9 c
10 d
11 a
12 d

GLOSSARY

abrasion A partial-thickness wound caused by the scraping away or rubbing of the skin

accountable Being responsible for one's actions and the actions of others who perform delegated tasks; answering questions about and explaining one's actions and the actions of others

air embolism Air that enters the cardiovascular system and travels to the lungs, where it obstructs blood flow

allergy A sensitivity to a substance that causes the body to react with signs and symptoms

antibody A substance in the blood plasma that fights or attacks (anti) antigens

antigen A substance that the body reacts to

apnea The lack or absence (a) of breathing (pnea)

arrhythmia Without (a) a rhythm

artifact Interference on the electrocardiogram

aspiration The breathing of fluid or an object into the lungs

Biot's respirations Irregular breathing with periods of apnea; respirations may be slow and deep or rapid and shallow

blood transfusion The intravenous administration of blood or its products

bradypnea Slow (brady) breathing (pnea); the respiratory rate is fewer than 10 respirations per minute

callus A thick, hardened area on the skin

catheter A tube used to drain or inject fluid through a body opening

catheterization The process of inserting a catheter

Cheyne-Stokes A breathing pattern in which respirations gradually increase in rate and depth and then become shallow and slow; breathing may stop (apnea) for 10 to 20 seconds

chronic wound A wound that does not heal easily

clean-contaminated wound A wound occurring from the surgical entry of the urinary, reproductive, respiratory, or gastrointestinal system

clean wound A wound that is not infected

closed wound A wound in which tissues are injured but the skin is not broken

confidentiality Trusting others with personal and private information

contaminated wound A wound with a high risk of infection

contamination The process by which an object or area becomes unclean

contusion A closed wound caused by a blow to the body

courtesy A polite, considerate, or helpful comment or act

dehiscence The separation of wound layers

delegate Authorizing another person to perform a task

dirty wound An infected wound

dyspnea Difficult, labored, or painful (dys) breathing (pnea)

dysrhythmia An abnormal (dys) rhythm

dysuria Difficult (dys) urination (uria)

electrocardiogram A recording (gram) of the electrical activity (electro) of the heart (cardio); ECG or EKG

electrocardiograph An instrument (graph) that records the electrical activity (electro) of the heart (cardio)

enteral nutrition Giving nutrients through the gastrointestinal tract (enteral)

erythrocyte Red (erythro) blood cell (cyte); carries oxygen to the cells

evisceration The separation of the wound along with the protrusion of abdominal organs

flow rate The number of drops per minute (gtt/min)

full-thickness wound The dermis, epidermis, and subcutaneous tissue are penetrated; muscle and bone may be involved

gastrostomy An opening (stomy) into the stomach (gastro)

gossip Spreading rumors or talking about the private matters of others

harassment Troubling, tormenting, offending, or worrying a person by one's behavior or comments

hematology The study (ology) of blood (hemat)

hematoma The collection of blood under the skin and tissues; a swelling (oma) that contains blood (hemat)

hematuria Blood (hemat) in the urine (uria)

hemoglobin The substance in red blood cells that picks up oxygen in the lungs and carries it to the cells; it gives blood its red color

hemolysis The destruction *(lysis)* of blood *(hemo)*

hemoptysis Bloody *(hemo)* sputum *(ptysis* meaning "to spit")

hemothorax The collection of blood *(hemo)* in the pleural space *(thorax)*

hyperventilation Respirations that are rapid *(hyper)* and deeper than normal

hypoventilation Respirations that are slow *(hypo)*, shallow, and sometimes irregular

hypoxemia A reduced amount *(hypo)* of oxygen *(ox)* in the blood *(emia)*

hypoxia A deficiency *(hypo)* of oxygen in the cells *(oxia)*

incision An open wound with clean, straight edges; usually intentionally produced with a sharp instrument

infected wound A wound that contains large amounts of bacteria and that shows signs of infection; a dirty wound

intentional wound A wound created for therapy

intravenous (IV) therapy The administration of fluids into a vein; IV and IV infusion

irrigation The process of washing out, flushing out, clearing, or cleaning a tube or body cavity

jejunostomy An opening *(stomy)* into the middle part of the small intestine *(jejuno)*

Kussmaul's respirations Very deep and rapid respirations; a sign of diabetic coma

laceration An open wound with torn tissues and jagged edges

lancet A short, disposable blade

lead A pair of electrodes; electrical activity is recorded between the electrodes

leukocyte White *(leuko)* blood cell *(cyte)*; protects the body against infection

meniscus The curved surface of a column of liquid

nasogastric (NG) tube A tube inserted through the nose *(naso)* into the stomach *(gastro)*

nasointestinal tube A tube inserted through the nose into the duodenum or jejunum of the small intestine

nonpathogen A microorganism that does not usually cause an infection

normal flora Microorganisms that usually live and grow in a certain location

open wound The skin or mucous membrane is broken

orthopnea Being able to breathe *(pnea)* deeply and comfortably only while sitting or standing *(ortho)*

orthopneic position Sitting up in bed *(ortho)* and leaning forward over the bedside table

oxygen concentration The amount of hemoglobin that contains oxygen (O_2)

palpate To feel or touch using your hands or fingers

partial-thickness wound A wound in which the dermis and epidermis of the skin are broken

pathogen A microorganism that causes an infection and is harmful

penetrating wound An open wound in which the skin and underlying tissues are pierced

percutaneous endoscopic gastrostomy (PEG) tube A tube inserted into the stomach *(gastro)* through a stab or puncture wound *(stomy)* made through *(per)* the skin *(cutaneous)*; a lighted instrument *(scope)* allows the doctor to see inside a body cavity or organ *(endo)*

phlebitis Inflammation *(itis)* of a vein *(phleb)*

plasma The liquid portion of the blood; it carries blood cells to other body cells

platelet Thrombocyte

pleural effusion The escape and collection of fluid (effusion) in the plueral space

pneumothorax The collection of air *(pneumo)* in the pleural space *(thorax)*

pollutant A harmful chemical or substance in the air or water

preceptor A teacher

puncture wound An open wound made by a sharp object; entry of the skin and underlying tissues may be intentional or unintentional

purulent drainage Thick, green, yellow, or brown drainage

red blood cells (RBCs) Erythrocytes

regurgitation The backward flow of food from the stomach into the mouth

residual urine The amount of urine left in the bladder after voiding

respiratory arrest Breathing stops

respiratory depression Slow, weak respirations that occur at a rate of fewer than 12 per minute; respirations are not deep enough to bring enough air into the lungs

responsibility The duty or obligation to perform some act or function

sanguineous drainage Bloody drainage *(sanguis)*

serosanguineous drainage Thin, watery drainage *(sero)* that is blood-tinged *(sanguineous)*

serous drainage Clear, watery fluid *(serum)*

sputum Expectorated mucus

sterile The absence of all microorganisms

sterile field A work area free of all pathogens and non-pathogens

sterile technique Surgical asepsis

suction The process of withdrawing or sucking up fluid (secretions)

surgical asepsis The practices that keep equipment and supplies free of all microorganisms; sterile technique

tachypnea Rapid *(tachy)* breathing *(pnea)*; the respiratory rate is usually more than 24 respirations per minute

task A function, procedure, activity, or work that does not require professional knowledge or judgment

thrombocyte A cell *(cyte)* necessary for the clotting *(thrombo)* of blood

tourniquet A constricting device applied to a limb to control bleeding

trauma An accident or violent act that injures the skin, mucous membranes, bones, and internal organs

unintentional wound A wound resulting from trauma

venipuncture A technique in which a vein *(veni)* is punctured

white blood cells (WBCs) Leukocytes

work ethics Behavior in the workplace

wound A break in the skin or mucous membrane

Index